Practical Microscopic Hematology

A Manual for the Clinical Laboratory and Clinical Practice

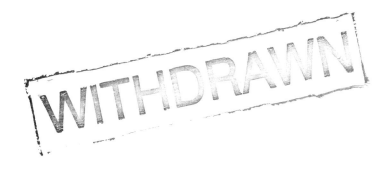

Practical Microscopic Hematology

A Manual for the Clinical Laboratory and Clinical Practice

Fritz Heckner, M.D.
Chief, Department of Medicine
Director, Clinical Hematology
Einbeck Hospital, Einbeck

H. Peter Lehmann, Ph.D.
and
Yuan S. Kao, M.D.
Department of Pathology
Louisiana State University Medical Center
New Orleans

Fourth English Edition

Lea & Febiger
PHILADELPHIA · BALTIMORE · HONG KONG
LONDON · MUNICH · SYDNEY · TOKYO
A WAVERLY COMPANY

Williams & Wilkins
Rose Tree Corporate Center, Building II
1400 North Providence Road, Suite 5025
Media, PA 19063-2043 USA

Executive Editor—J. Matthew Harris
Development Editor—Lisa Stead
Project/Manuscript Editor—Jessica Howie Martin/Karen Cuzzolino
Production Manager—Samuel A. Rondinelli

Library of Congress Cataloging-in-Publication Data

Heckner, Fritz.
    [Praktikum der mikroscopischen Hämatologie. English]
    Practical microscopic hematology : a manual for the
clinical laboratory and clinical practice / Fritz Heckner ; [edited
by] H. Peter Lehmann and Yuan S. Kao. — 4th English ed.
      p.   cm.
    Updated translation of: Praktikum der mikroscopischen Hämatologie. 7th ed.
    Includes index.
    ISBN 0-8121-1711-5. — ISBN 3-541-70813-1
    1. Blood cells—Atlases. 2. Hematology—Atlases. 3. Medical
microscopy—Atlases. I. Lehmann, H. Peter (Hermann Peter), 1937–
II. Kao, Yuan S., 1935–   III. Title.
    [DNLM: 1. Blood Cells—atlases. WH 17 H449L 1933a]
RB45.H39813   1993
616.07'561—dc20
DNLM/DLC
for Library of Congress   93-23016
                                                   CIP

First edition 1980:   ISBN 0-8067-0811-5 (Baltimore)
                     ISBN 3-541-70811-5 (München)
Second edition 1982: ISBN 0-8067-0812-3 (Baltimore)
                     ISBN 3-541-70812-3 (München)
Third edition 1988: ISBN 0-8067-0813-1 (Baltimore)
                     ISBN 3-541-70813-1 (München)
All rights including that of translation, reserved. No part of this publication may be reproduced, stored in a retrieval system, or transmitted in any other form or by any means, electronic, mechanical, recording or otherwise without the prior written permission of the publisher.

Printed in Germany by Kastner & Callwey, München

NOTE: Although the author(s) and the publisher have taken reasonable steps to ensure the accuracy of the drug information included in this text before publication, drug information may change without notice and readers are advised to consult the manufacturer's packaging inserts before prescribing medications.

PRINTED IN THE UNITED STATES OF AMERICA

Print number: 5   4   3

Preface

Although automated analysis procedures are an increasingly important component of the clinical hematology laboratory, morphologic examination of the blood and bone marrow cells remains a significant and crucial diagnostic tool.

The aim of *Practical Microscopic Hematology* remains the same as that of the first edition: namely, to assist clinicians, laboratory technicians, and students in the differentiation and interpretation of blood and bone marrow smears under microscopic examination. The fourth English edition contains the changes made by Professor Heckner in preparing the seventh German edition: clarification of the FAB classification of myelodysplastic syndrome and the Kiel classification of non-Hodgkin's lymphoma and the significance of monoclonal antibodies in diagnostic hematology. Also, some new photographs have been added and some have been replaced to clarify certain sections.

As with the earlier editions, we thank Professor Heckner for his support and the technical staff at Lea & Febiger for their assistance and cooperation in the preparation of this book.

New Orleans, Louisiana
March 1993

H. Peter Lehmann
Yuan S. Kao

Preface to the First English Edition

The diagnosis of blood disorders depends to a large extent on the microscopic examination of blood or bone marrow smears. While automation in the clinical hematology laboratory has revolutionized cell-counting procedures, it has not, to date, superseded visual inspection of smears under the microscope. The present manual is intended to assist clinicians, laboratory technicians and students in the differentiation and interpretation of blood and bone marrow smears under microscopic examination. For this purpose a description of normal blood and bone marrow cells is given along with photomicrographs of typical cells and cellular elements. Illustrations of blood and bone marrow in diseases are given, with brief explanations for guidance in interpretation. The text gives only such information considered necessary for an understanding of the illustrations. Discussions of the diseases illustrated and literature sources are intentionally omitted, because the book is intended to be a manual to assist in microscopic examinations and not a comprehensive text in hematology.

We have adhered strictly to the format used by Professor Heckner in the 4th German edition of Praktikum der mikroskopischen Hämatologie, substituting American terminology where appropriate. All the illustrations are those used by Professor Heckner in the 4th edition of his book. That the book has now appeared in four German editions, since the first in 1965, indicates the need for such a manual, at least in the German-speaking countries. It is our hope that this English edition will be useful to persons working in hematology, as well as students learning hematology in English-speaking countries.

We are grateful to Professor Heckner for the freedom he has allowed us in the preparation of this book. It is our hope that we have been able to retain the sense and clarity of his descriptions for the English edition. We should like to express our appreciation to Dr. Hans Leo Lehmann for the translation of the 4th German Edition, and to Ms. Kathy Fisher for typing the manuscript. Finally, we thank the publisher, Urban & Schwarzenberg, for the continual help and cooperation we have received while preparing this book.

New Orleans, Louisiana
September, 1979

H. Peter Lehmann
Yuan S. Kao

Contents

1 Technical Introduction

In many institutions, the determination of the blood differential on automated instrumentation has replaced visual examination of cytomorphologic structures of blood cells. Although even abnormal cell structures are registered on these instruments, they are not recognized qualitatively, thus ensuring a place for visual microscopic examination of blood cells in the hematologic diagnostic process. Additionally, in small institutions and physicians' office laboratories, automated instrumentation for the determination of the leukocyte differential is often not available. Therefore, a description of the preparation and staining of blood and bone marrow smears is still appropriate.

1.1   Smear Preparation

Naturally, the technical expertise necessary to make good blood and bone marrow smears cannot be learned from a book, but can only be acquired by practical experience. On the other hand, reliable evaluation of cell preparations depends, to a large extent, on the quality of the smears and on their appropriate staining. For this reason, some instruction on smear preparation will be given to avoid production of poor slides.

Good smear preparation requires the use of scrupulously clean slides; otherwise, smears with uneven or unsatisfactory staining are often obtained. At one time, glass slides were treated with a chromic-sulphuric acid mixture, followed by thorough rinsing with distilled water, to achieve the necessary cleanliness prior to use. Now, however, commercially prepared slides are available, some with a ground section for marking, that do not require any special pretreatment. All slides must be kept free from dust, and a sufficiently large stock should always be on hand.

In the preparation of blood smears, which can be made with the ground edge of a coverglass or with a smooth-edge slide, care must be taken to ensure that no more than two thirds to three quarters of the slide is taken up by the smear. The smearing technique must be such that in the final film some of the erythrocytes lie separated side by side, and some are aggregated in small rouleaux. Smears that are too thick result in overstaining and, because the individual cells are not spread out sufficiently, make the microscopic analysis of the cellular fine structure impossible. The acquisition of a good smearing technique, therefore, is essential, and is only possible through a great deal of practice.

Bone marrow smears can be prepared in the same way as blood smears. The aspirated marrow, with or without anticoagulant, is collected in a large Petri dish, and the surplus marrow blood is drained off by inclining the dish. Several small portions of marrow fluid containing granulated particles are collected from the bottom of the Petri dish, with a transfer pipet, for the smear. The smear prepared in this way should contain numerous small marrow particles. Three or four more slides should be prepared by squeezing isolated marrow particles, which have been separated from the aspirated marrow with the edge of a slide or with a small wooden stick. If only a few marrow particles are available, the squeezed particle smear should be used exclusively. Care must be taken in squeezing the marrow particles to preserve the cells. This can be done by drawing a second slide longitudinally over the first slide under gentle pressure, thereby spreading the particulate material into a thin layer. Reliable microscopic examination requires that smears of bone marrow aspirates contain sufficiently thin areas of evenly distributed, intact, and closely packed cell elements. Generally, thick marrow smears are not suitable for morphologic diagnosis.

Staining of the blood and bone marrow smears should be individually adapted to certain standard staining procedures. The most widely used staining procedure (Wright/ Pappenheim) begins with the application of the May-Grünwald stain for a short time (4 to 6 minutes), resulting in the simultaneous alcohol-fixation of the specimen. The specimens should then be rinsed with distilled water. The subsequent staining conditions (concentration of stain and time of staining) with dilute Giemsa solution should be adapted to the requirements of the individual laboratory. The critical factor in the staining is the pH of the distilled water, which should be as close to pH 7.0 as possible. This requirement may be difficult to achieve in practice, but it need not be detrimental to the staining process as long as large variations in pH are avoided. A longer staining time is used with a more acidic pH, and shorter times are used if the water is basic. If a satisfactory universal stain cannot be obtained in this way, buffering of the Giemsa solution as follows is recommended: 1 part Giemsa stock solution added to 20 parts 0.0667 mol/L phosphate buffer solution, pH 7.0 to 7.2. Alternatively, commercial Wright's stain (a methyl alcohol solution of eosin and a complex mixture of thiazines) may be used, with a buffer solution of pH 6.4. The staining time with this stain-buffer mixture is approximately 15 to 20 minutes. Finally, special attention should be paid to regular cleaning of the glassware used in the preparation of the Giemsa solution and to occasional filtering of the stock stain solutions. Special staining and cytochemical methods are described in the Appendix.

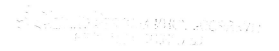

To obtain a preliminary indication of the quantity and quality of the cells, the routine microscopic examination of the smear specimen is initially carried out by scanning the slide under low- and high-power dry lenses. For this examination, the use of a thin coverglass is recommended to reduce light scattering from the surface of the smear. Many cytologic diagnoses can be made using the high-power dry lens, but for the assessment of erythrocyte morphology, an oil immersion lens must be used. The final differentiation of the cells in the blood smear should be carried out with an oil immersion lens. Microscopic examination should be made on the feather edge (the end third) of the smear; the tailings, however, should be disregarded because partly damaged white cell elements that may lead to false cell counts are artificially concentrated in this region. On the other hand, specific pathologic cells may be found in this region of slide, as well as at the edges of the smear. To accurately evaluate erythrocyte morphology, one must remember that the shape of the red blood cells may be altered in excessively thin or thick portions of the smear. Marrow aspirates should also first be examined using dry objectives to get a general view of the cell composition and to guard against missing localized areas of specific cells, such as groups of tumor cells or cells from granulomatous lesions. Any unusual findings must then be examined carefully under oil immersion. A combined microscopic examination of the marrow fluid as described is essential, and has almost the same significance as a count of at least 1000 cells. A combined qualitative and quantitative differentiation of bone marrow smears is usually not necessary, except for specific diagnostic purposes, for example, establishment of fraction of blast cells. All persons interested in hematology should have a collection of slides. The slides should be stored in a case, and should be carefully cleaned with soft cotton-wool or strips of muslin saturated with xylol or with commercially available lens cleaner to remove the immersion oil after each examination. This procedure prevents fading of the stain through the action of the immersion oil.

General Rule for Microscopic Hematology Diagnosis. Only an examination of a combination of blood and bone marrow smears makes a complete diagnosis possible.

1.2   Preparation of a Buffy Coat (Leukocyte Concentrate) Smear

Venous blood drawn into an EDTA Vacutainer® tube (liquid or powder) is recommended. (Sodium citrate Vacutainer tubes are also acceptable.) The tubes must be properly filled with blood and may stand for 2 to 3 hours after collection and still give acceptable smears. The contents of the tube must be carefully mixed and centrifuged for 15 minutes at 1500 rpm. After centrifugation and removal of the plasma (with a pipet), 0.3 to 0.5 ml of the buffy coat layer is drawn up into a finely drawn out pipet. A small amount of erythrocyte layer drawn up with the leukocytes does not affect the final examination. A few drops of leukocyte layer are then smeared onto microscopic slides, in the same way used for the whole blood smear, and are stained by the Pappenheim procedure or by other cytochemical methods (Fig. 1).

Indications for Use of a Buffy Coat Smear
1. Increased number of cells in leukopenia.
2. Examination for abnormal cells in leukopenia.
3. Cytochemical reactions in leukopenia.
4. Remission and relapse of acute leukemias.
5. Search for sex chromatin.

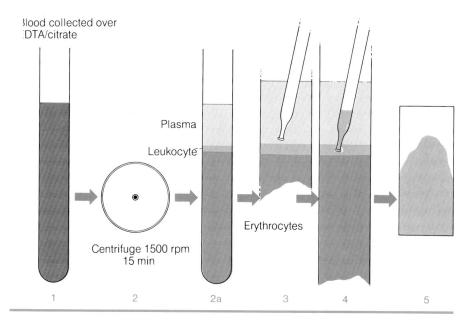

Blood collected over EDTA/citrate

Plasma

Leukocyte

Centrifuge 1500 rpm
15 min

Erythrocytes

1   2   2a   3   4   5

Fig. 1.   Preparation of a blood smear from the buffy coat (leukocyte concentrate).

Fig. 2. a, Schematic electron microscopic representation of the cell structures of a nucleated blood-forming cell. **(1)** Nucleus, rich in DNA, carrier of chromosomes; **(2)** nucleolus, rich in RNA; **(3)** cytoplasm, with RNA rich polyribosomes; **(4)** Golgi complex, with centrioles; **(5)** mitochondria; **(6)** specific granules (neutrophils, basophils, eosinophils); **(7)** vacuole; **(8)** lysosomes (e.g., azurophilic granulation); **(9)** polyribosomes, RNA carriers (only recognizable as plasma basophilia under light microscopy); **(10)** endoplasmic reticulum (rarely seen under light microscopy as discrete bright streaks in the cytoplasm, e.g., in plasma cells). **b,** Same cell schematic as in Figure 2a, fixed and stained, and seen under light microscopy and oil immersion, × 1000 (labeling as in Figure 2a). **(1–3)** Largely identical with electron microscopy; **(4)** light perinuclear zone (centrosphere); **(5)** small bright regions in the cytoplasm (lipid-containing mitochondria, dissolved on alcohol fixation); **(6)** forms that can still be differentiated (as in electron microscopy) through staining; **(7)** vacuoles under light microscopy (mostly fat droplets); **(8)** small red-violet granules.

2   Significant Intracellular Structures of a Nucleated Blood-Forming Cell

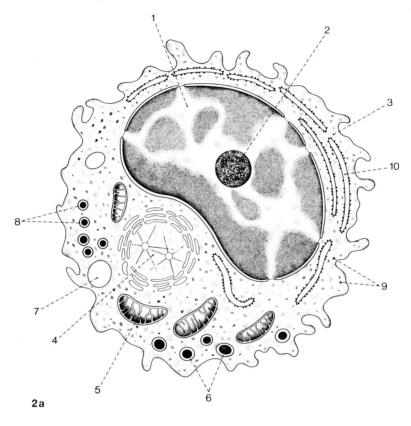

2a

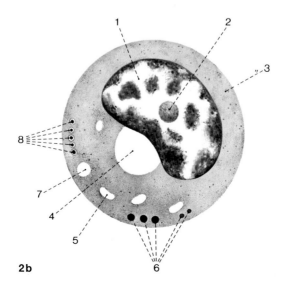

2b

Fig. 3. Schematic diagram of normal hematopoietic cell differentiation. **(1)** Pluripotent stem cell; **(2)** myelopoietic stem cell; **(3)** lymphopoietic stem cell; **(4–7)** committed stem cells of myelopoiesis (erythropoiesis, granulopoiesis, thrombopoiesis, and monocyte development); **(8)** precursor cell of B-lymphocytes (pre-B cell); **(9)** precursor cell of T-lymphocytes (pre-T cell). (Cell forms in the blue shaded area are not microscopically discernible.)

3 Normal Morphology of Blood and Bone Marrow Cells

3.1 Hematopoietic Cell Differentiation

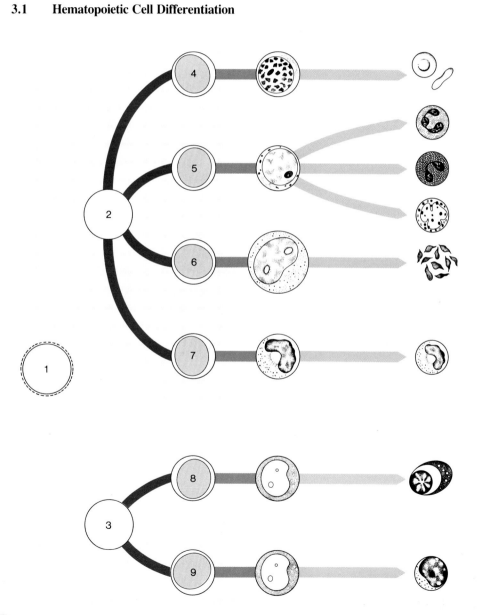

3.2   Erythropoiesis

3.2.1   Cells in the Development of Erythrocytes in the Bone Marrow

Pronormoblast (Proerythroblast) (Figs. 4a–c).   The most immature and, therefore, largest cell in erythropoiesis. The nucleus is round, stains dark violet, and has a densely packed and even chromatin structure with indistinct (blue) nucleoli. The cytoplasm is pale blue with spotty or sickle-shaped lighter areas (hyaloplasma), depending on the localization of the Golgi zone and the lipid-containing mitochondria. A tendency to mechanical damage causes plasma extrusions (earlets). In mitosis, sieve-like brightening caused by a diffuse distribution of the mitochondria occurs over the entire cytoplasm.

Macroblast (Macropronormoblast) (Figs. 4a, b).   Cell form resulting from the so-called hemiheteroplastic division of the pronormoblast, which it resembles morphologically and from which it is distinguished only by a smaller cell diameter. The composition of the nucleus may be of varying density, so that certain transitions to the cell types formed in the subsequent steps of erythropoiesis become noticeable.

Cells Formed by Maturation and Division

Basophilic Normoblast (Fig. 4d).   The cell diameter, compared to that of the macroblast, is further decreased. The nucleus is round and contains characteristically checked chromatin with strong contrasts—light-colored farrows between dark-violet chromatin particles (also described, incorrectly, as "spoke wheel structure"). The cytoplasm is moderately basophilic.

Polychromatic Normoblast (Fig. 4e).   The shape of the cell and structure of the nucleus are similar to those of the basophilic normoblast, but the cell diameter is further decreased. The cytoplasm is blue-gray-violet (a mixed coloration caused by progressive production of hemoglobin–incipient acidophilia).

Orthochromatic Normoblast (Acidophil) (Fig. 4f).   In this cell group, there has been further progressive reduction in the size of the nucleus, with a corresponding increase in density of the chromatin (pyknosis), which may be seen as a homogeneous black residual structure. The cytoplasm is a gray-yellow-red at the outer edge, which is often not clearly defined. At this stage of erythrocyte development, synthesis of hemoglobin is complete.

Disappearance of the Nucleus of the Normoblast, and Maturation Toward the Non-nucleated Red Cell Elements in Peripheral Blood

Appearance of So-called Basophilic Substances in the Erythrocytes

Reticulocyte (Fig. 5a).   Characterized by the presence of granular or reticular filamentous structures in about 0.5 to 1.5% of all erythrocytes. These structures are discernible only

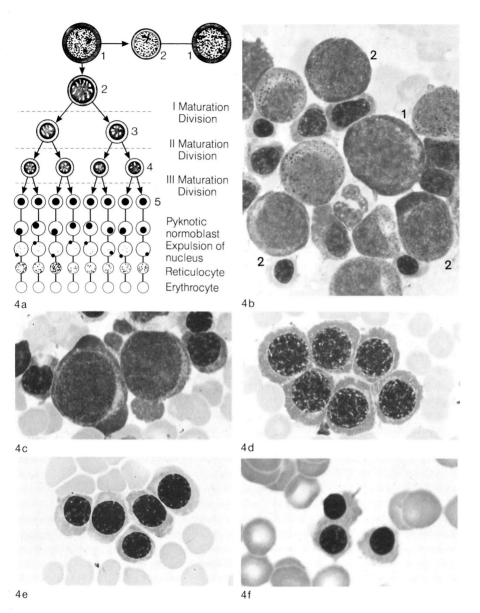

I Maturation
Division

II Maturation
Division

III Maturation
Division

Pyknotic
normoblast
Expulsion of
nucleus
Reticulocyte
Erythrocyte

4a

4b

4c

4d

4e

4f

Fig. 4. Erythropoiesis. **a,** Erythron stem line of erythropoietic cells (1–5). **b,** Pronormoblast (1) and macroblast (2). **c,** Pronormoblasts with typical cytoplasmic extrusions. **d,** Basophilic normoblast. **e,** Polychromatic normoblast. **f,** Orthochromatic normoblast, partly with early nuclear pyknosis. Note: The numbers alongside the individual cell types correspond to the arabic numbers in Figure 4a.

after staining with methylene blue, when erythrocytes are a pale greenish-blue and the filamentous structure is blue-black. In pathologic conditions, such as hemolytic anemia or acute blood loss, reticulocytosis becomes prominent. A pathologic variant is the achromoreticulocyte (see "Hemolytic Anemia"), which contains reticular filamentous structures without visible cell bodies.

Morphologic Equivalents of the Reticulocyte

Polychromasia (Fig. 5b).   The violet tinting seen in some erythrocytes after Giemsa or Wright's staining corresponds to the appearance of extremely find basophilic stippling. Thus this is also a regeneration (increased erythropoiesis) phenomenon. The basophilic substances in the basophilic-stippled erythrocytes and in polychromasia (see also sections 6 and 8) are RNA-containing remnants (ribosomes) of the cytoplasm of the proerythroblasts. Polychromatic erythrocytes (reticulocytes) are always larger than normocytes, and their cell membranes are slightly folded or indented.

Basophilic Stippling of the Erythrocyte (Fig. 5c).   Seen as an extremely fine blue-black stippling diffusely distributed in the cell. It is recognizable only with conventional Giemsa or Wright's staining, or with special staining by the Manson-Schwartz procedure, using a basic 1% methylene blue solution. Basophilic-stippled erythrocytes are rarely found in normal blood. Increased occurrence always corresponds to reticulocytosis, and is evidence of increased erythropoiesis or disturbance of hemoglobin synthesis [see "Hemolytic Anemia," Fig. 37g (lead poisoning)]. The basophilic stippling corresponds to RNA-containing aggregated ribosomes and is formed during the drying of the blood smear.

End Product of Erythropoiesis

Erythrocyte (Normocyte) (Fig. 5d).   Reddish, circular, biconcave cells; all cells have almost the same size (diameter 7 to 8 μm) and no visible internal structure. The brightness in the center of the cell is caused by its biconcave disk shape.

Other Internal Structures of Erythrocytes

Jolly Bodies (Howell-Jolly Bodies) (Fig. 5e).   DNA-containing pyknotic nuclear remnants seen in erythrocytes on Wright's staining. Increased in number in hyposplenism, following splenectomy, in hemolytic anemia, and in megaloblastic anemia.

Cabot's Rings (Fig. 5f).   Pathologic loop-shaped occlusion found in erythrocytes during failure of erythropoiesis or in extramedullary blood formation. (Formed from a remnant of the nuclear membrane or from part of a mitotic spindle.)

Sideroblast (physiologic) (Fig. 5g).   Normoblast (20 to 60% of total) containing ferritin molecules (as many as 5 are normal); also called siderosome. These cells are absent in iron deficiency anemia and in anemia resulting from infection.

Siderocyte (Fig. 5h).   Normal reticulocyte that contains iron (hemosiderin or ferritin) in the mitochondria. These cells have no diagnostic significance.

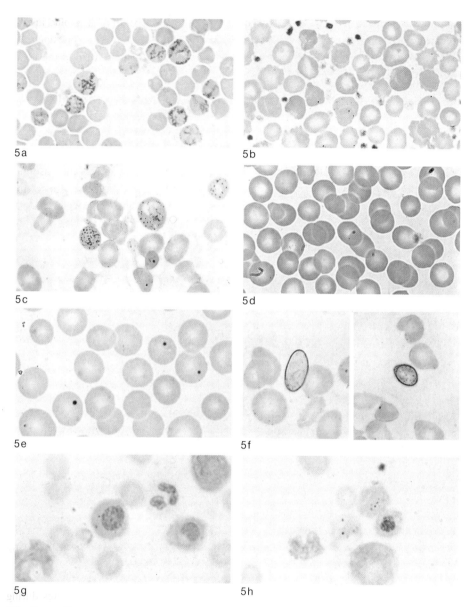

Fig. 5. **a,** Supravital stain showing multiple reticulocytes. **b,** Polychromasia of erythrocytes (also note thrombocytosis). **c,** Basophilic stippling of erythrocyte (punctate basophilia). **d,** Normal erythrocytes. **e,** Howell-Jolly bodies in erythrocytes (Wright's stain). **f,** Cabot's ring and "fine" chromatin dust in the erythrocyte. **g,** Sideroblast. **h,** Siderocyte.

3.2.2   Basic Rules for Erythropoiesis

Cells, and especially nuclei, are always round.

Cytoplasmic basophilia (caused by the presence of ribonucleic acid) is an indication of cell immaturity and lack of hemoglobin.

Cytoplasmic acidophilia (caused by the presence of hemoglobin) is an indication of cell maturity.

The cytoplasm of the erythrocyte precursors (containing a nucleus) never contains specific granulation.

Basophilic stippling of the erythrocytes and polychromasia are identical cell characteristics, and are evidence of regenerating or pseudoregenerating erythropoiesis or of a disturbance in hemoglobin synthesis.

Nucleus-containing red cell elements are not a physiologic component of the peripheral blood (blood smear).

3.3   Granulopoiesis

3.3.1   Cells in the Development of Granulocytes (Leukocytes) in Bone Marrow

Myeloblast (Figs. 6a–b; 9).   The least mature cell form of granulopoiesis. It is only sparsely present in the bone marrow, and has a cell diameter slightly smaller than that of the proerythroblast. The myeloblast exists in various cell shapes, and has a nucleus that is often oval and is slightly indented on one side. The chromatin is in fine, closely meshed, transparent filaments. Nucleoli (two to five), which may coalesce, are clearly visible. The cytoplasm is small, is moderately to weakly basophilic, and contains a faint perinuclear lighter zone. Type I: without granulation (Fig. 6a–c); Type II: with incipient granulation (Fig. 6d).

Promyelocyte (Figs. 7a–d).   A cell group consisting of diverse elements that are particularly variable in their nuclear-to-cytoplasmic ratio and in their degree of granulation. Some common promyelocyte characteristics are an oval-shaped nucleus, often flattened or indented on one side (kidney shaped); medium-density chromatin; and inhomogeneous reticulations. Nucleoli are often visible. The cytoplasm is a medium to light blue, with a small irregular-shaped lighter zone in the vicinity of the indentation of the nucleus (centrosphere), and contains azurophilic (red-violet) granules.

Early Promyelocyte (Fig. 7a–d).   This is the most frequent cell type of immature granulopoiesis. The earliest forms still show a close morphologic relationship to the myeloblast. Often the nucleus contains visible nucleoli, and the cytoplasm clearly shows a few azurophilic granules. The fully developed early promyelocyte is the largest cell of the granulocyte series because of the increase in size of the cytoplasm. It contains many azurophilic granules, some with a coarser grain than others. Occasionally, plasma fragments with typical granulations are visible (see Fig. 2b, no. 4).

Cells Formed by Division During Maturation

Late Promyelocyte or Semimature Myelocyte (Figs. 8a; 9).   This cell has a smaller diameter, fewer nucleoli, a less basophilic cytoplasm, and less azurophilic granulation than does the early promyelocyte. Occasionally, the cytoplasm begins to take on the coloration of the myelocyte.

Myelocyte, Neutrophil (First Evidence of Specific Granulation) (Figs. 8b; 9).   The neutrophil shows a further decrease in the cell diameter and in the size of the nucleus. The chromatin

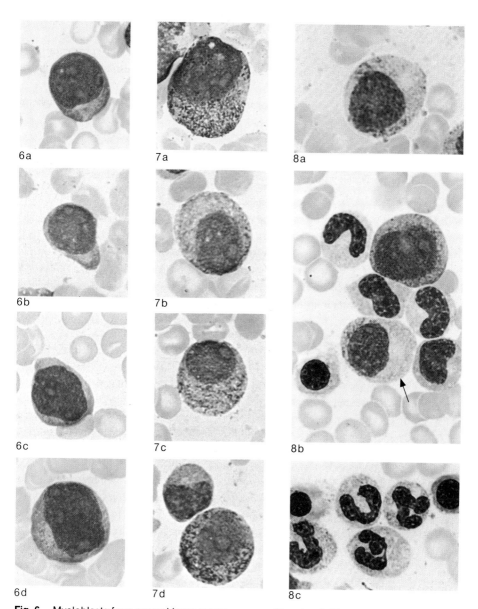

Fig. 6. Myeloblasts from normal bone marrow. **a–c,** Type I. **d,** Type II.

Fig. 7. Various shapes of promyelocytes. **b,** Small amount of azurogranulation. **c,** Late promyelocyte with prominent cytoplasmic granules.

Fig. 8. a, Late promyelocyte. **b,** Promelocyte, neutrophil myelocyte (arrow), three neutrophil metamyelocytes, one band cell, and one normoblast (lower left corner). **c,** Two neutrophil bands and two segmented neutrophils.

structure becomes more coarse, and nucleoli are only rarely visible. The cytoplasm is no longer basophilic and takes on a pale gray-brown or pink-brown color. The cells show the first appearance of specific granulation—fine brownish-violet (neutrophilic) granules taking the place of the azurophilic granulation found in the promyelocytes. Also, a characteristic prominent light spot is in the area of the deeper nuclear indentation (centrosphere).

End of the Maturation Divisions

Further cell development is by maturation of the nucleus.

Metamyelocyte, Neutrophil (Figs. 8b; 9).   The cell nucleus is transformed into the characteristic bean or kidney shape, and the chromatin is coarse and compacted in spots, especially at both poles. The cytoplasm is similar to that seen in the neutrophilic myelocyte but without the centrosphere.

Physiologic Cell Migration into Peripheral Blood

Granulocyte (Leukocyte) with Band-form Nucleus, Band Neutrophil (Fig. 8b–c).   Narrowing of the nucleus has taken place, thereby forming a C- or S-shaped nucleus without recognizable compression farrows (ribbon shaped). A further coarsening of the chromatin particles (leopard-skin pattern) has also occurred. Otherwise, the neutrophilic band cell resembles the metamyelocyte.

Granulocyte (Leukocyte) with Segmented Nucleus, Neutrophilic Granulocyte, Segmented Neutrophil, Polymorphonuclear Leukocyte (Figs. 8c, 10).   These cells are mature leukocytes. In most cases, the nucleus is made up of three to five segments connected by filaments. A filament is defined as a thread-like connection between lobes of the nucleus that is so narrow that it contains no significant, or visible, nuclear material. The nuclear chromatin and cytoplasm of segmented neutrophils are similar to those of a band neutrophil. Occasionally, the segmented lobes are superimposed and no filament is visible. In case of doubt during examination of the blood smear, the cell should be called a segmented neutrophil rather than a band neutrophil.

3.3.2   Sex-Specific Structures on the Nucleus of Granulocytes (Fig. 11)

The (so-called) sex-specific structures (sex chromatin) attached to the granulocyte nucleus are:

Drumstick: presence of at least 6 per 500 granulocytes is proof of female sex.
Sessile nodule: early stage of drumstick in female.
Small club: not specific, found more frequently in male.
Racket: not specific (rare).

3.3.3   Development of Eosinophilic Granulocytes (Eosinophils)

Eosinophilic Blast, Eosinophiloblast.   Under physiologic conditions, not unambiguously definable in bone marrow.

Eosinophilic Promyelocyte (Figs. 12a; 13a).   Has the typical characteristics of a promyelocyte in addition to deposition of eosinophilic granules in the cytoplasm. These granules,

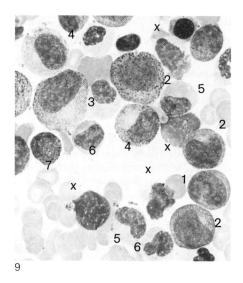

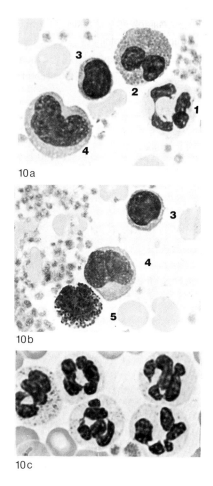

Fig. 9. Normal granulopoiesis in the bone marrow (×750). **(1)** Myeloblast; **(2)** early promyelocyte; **(3)** late promyelocyte; **(4) neutrophilic myelocyte; (5)** neutrophilic metamyelocyte; **(6)** transition to band form; **(7)** eosinophilic band form; **(x)** artifacts—nuclear debris.

Fig. 10. a,b, Normal cells in blood smear. **(1)** Granulocyte (with a segmented nucleus); **(2)** eosinophils; **(3)** lymphocyte; **(4)** monocytes; **(5)** basophils (with numerous thrombocytes close by). **c,** Neutrophilic granulocyte, hypersegmented nucleus (shift to the right).

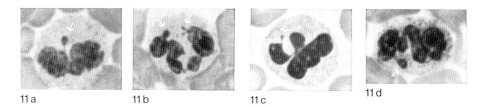

Fig. 11. Sex-specific (sex chromatin) and nonspecific appendages of the segmented neutrophils (arrows). **a,** Drumstick. **b,** Sessile nodule (left), small clubs (right). **c,** Small club. **d,** Racket.

in sufficient numbers, may obscure the azurophilic granulation. Depending on the staining conditions (pH of the Giemsa solution), the eosinophilic granules appear as black-gray, gray-brown, rust-colored, or brick-red small spheres, which occasionally also cover the nucleus. The black-gray granules (which can be confused with basophilic granules) are less mature than the reddish granules and, therefore, are only seen in the precursors of the eosinophilic leukocytes.

Eosinophilic Myelocyte (Figs. 12b; 13b).   Seen more frequently than the eosinophilic pro-myelocyte in bone marrow. The appearance of the nucleus and the nuclear-to-cytoplasmic ratio are similar to those of the neutrophilic myelocyte. The cytoplasm is full of eosinophilic granules, which are predominantly brown-red or reddish. Areas of the cytoplasm not covered by granules show slight basophilia.

Eosinophilic Metamyelocyte (Figs. 12c; 13c) and **Eosinophilic Leukocyte with Band Nucleus.** Because of the rapid maturation of the nucleus, these two cell classes are not usually separated. Morphologically, they are similar to the equivalent forms of the neutrophil series, but contain mature eosinophilic granules.

Eosinophilic Leukocyte with Segmented Nucleus (Figs. 13d; 14).   This most mature cell form of eosinophilic granulopoiesis is capable of migration into the peripheral blood. The nucleus is predominantly double segmented with a finely filamentous bridge. The chromatin is coarse and, in the center of the segment, stands out in spots. The cytoplasm is almost completely filled with mature eosinophilic granules of different sizes. The bright basophilic color of the cytoplasm can be seen only in areas not covered by granules.

3.3.4   Development of Basophilic Granulocytes (Basophils)

Basophiloblast (Basophilic Myeloblast) (Fig. 15a).   Cell with a myeloblast-like nucleus with chromatin of variable density. This cell is rarely seen in bone marrow. The nucleoli are indistinct or not visible. The cytoplasm is moderately large and contains a few dark-violet (basophilic) granules of varying size, which sometimes also cover the cell nucleus. Also present are small vacuoles arising from leached-out granules. The cell rarely divides.

Minimal Differentiated Maturation of the Nucleus without Formation of Typical Myelocytic Intermediate Forms

Basophilic Granulocyte (Basophilic Leukocyte) (Fig. 15b–d).   Cell form with little sign of maturation. Most of the nuclei are only indented in several places (cloverleaf form) or are roughly segmented. The chromatin is moderately spotted and not markedly lumpy. The nucleus is partly covered by the basophilic granules. The cytoplasm is relatively narrow and loosely permeated by intensely basophilic granules, which often form a wreath-like peripheral area. The basic color of the cytoplasm is pale blue to pale pink. Vacuoles caused by degranulation are often seen.

3.3.5   Development of Monocytes

Monoblast.   Found in normal bone marrow; not readily distinguishable from the myelo-blast.

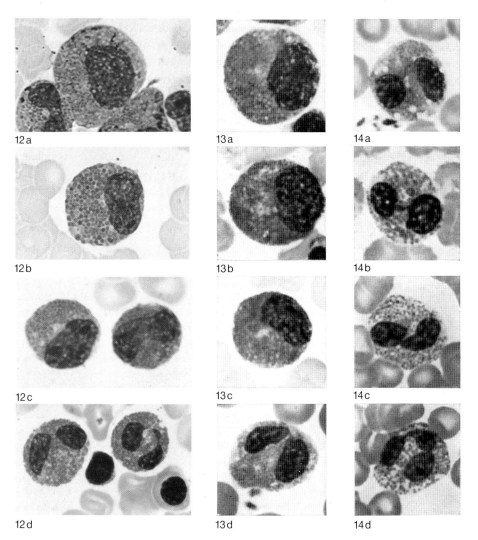

12a   13a   14a

12b   13b   14b

12c   13c   14c

12d   13d   14d

Fig. 12. **a,** Eosinophilic promyelocyte. **b,** Eosinophilic myelocyte (stained under slightly acid conditions). **c,** Two eosinophilic metamyelocytes. **d,** Two eosinophilic leukocytes.

Fig. 13. **a,** Eosinophilic promyelocyte. **b,** Eosinophilic myelocyte. **c,** Eosinophilic metamyelocyte. **d,** Eosinophilic leukocyte with segmented nucleus.

Fig. 14. Eosinophilic segmented leukocytes. **b,** The nuclear form corresponds to a racket. **d,** A third segment is present.

Promonocyte (reliable differentiation by cytochemical techniques—nonspecific esterase) (Fig. 16b).   A large cell, found only in the bone marrow, that has predominantly promyelocytic characteristics. The nucleus has unilateral, sometimes irregular, indentation; fine chromatin in coarse filaments and isolated nucleoli are visible. The cytoplasm is light basophilic with a small centrosphere and contains azurophilic granules. The transitions to the next cell type are indistinct. Both promonocyte and monocyte can be identified.

Monocyte (Figs. 16c; 17).   The largest cell found in the peripheral blood. The nucleus is large, characteristically lobulated, and may also be bean shaped. The chromatin is generally loose and coarsely filamentous, and may have some dense areas. There are no recognizable nucleoli, and the staining is less dense than that in the lymphocyte. The cytoplasm is lightly basophilic or a gray-blue color, and often appears dusted with azurophilic granules.

3.3.6   Basic Rules for Granulopoiesis

Myeloblast: the only cell of the leukocyte series with no granulation. Type I: most immature morphologically distinguishable cell of granulopoiesis. Type II: first recognizable azurophilic granulation.

Four distinct forms of granulation are found in the following cells:
a. Azurophilic granulation: Type II myeloblasts, promyelocytes, promonocytes, and monocytes.
b. Neutrophilic granulation: neutrophilic myelocytes, metamyelocytes with rod-shaped and segmented nuclei.
c. Eosinophilic granulation: eosinophilic promyelocytes, myelocytes, metamyelocytes with band and segmented nuclei.
d. Basophilic granulation: basophiloblasts and basophilic granulocytes.

The shape of the nucleus changes with cell development; the degree of differentiation of the nucleus decreases from the neutrophils to the basophils.

Morphologic definition of the neutrophil:
a. Neutrophilic myelocyte: neutrophilic granulocyte with mature cytoplasm and a round or oval nucleus. The ratio of the axes of an oval nucleus should not be more than $1:2$.
b. Neutrophilic metamyelocyte (synonym—juvenile): neutrophilic granulocyte with mature cytoplasm and kidney-shaped nucleus. The indentation of the nucleus should not be more than half the shorter diameter of the nucleus if it were oval shaped.
c. Neutrophilic granulocyte with band-shaped nucleus (band, stab, neutrophilic band): neutrophilic granulocyte with mature cytoplasm and a horseshoe-shaped or S-shaped nucleus. The nucleus shows a clearly recognizable ribbon shape. The diameter of the narrowest part of the nucleus must be greater than one third of the diameter of the thickest part of the nucleus.
d. Neutrophilic granulocyte with polymorphous nucleus; polymorphonuclear leukocyte (synonyms—segmented neutrophil, filament-nucleated neutrophil, PMN): neutrophilic granulocyte with a mature cytoplasm. The nucleus either clearly shows at least two and possibly three or more segments or does not fit the nuclear description previously given for the myelocyte, metamyelocyte, or band.

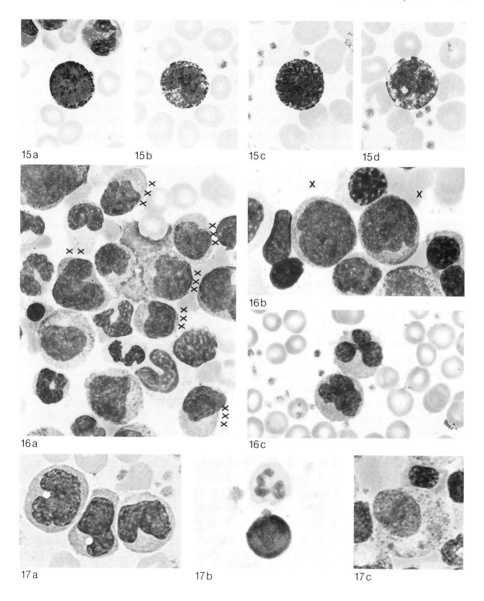

15a   15b   15c   15d

16b

16a   16c

17a   17b   17c

Fig. 15. **a,** Basophiloblast. **b–c,** Basophilic leukocytes. **d,** Basophilic leukocyte shows loss of granules.

Fig. 16. Monocyte formation. **a,** Promonocyte **(XX)**; mature monocyte **(XXX)**. **b,** Immature promonocytes **(X).** **c,** Various types of monocytes.

Fig. 17. **a,** Typical monocytes seen in peripheral blood. **b,** Positive nonspecific esterase reaction in a monocyte, and a negative reaction of a granulocyte. **c,** Histiocytic functional form of the monocyte (i.e., macrophage) in the bone marrow.

Leukocyte composition of the peripheral blood (white blood cell differential—WBC):

a. Total leukocyte count: $4.0 - 10.0 \times 10^9$/L

b. Differential:

Cell Type	Percent	Range of Absolute Counts $\times 10^9$/L
Basophils	0–1	0.00–0.09
Eosinophils	1–4	0.04–0.36
Band neutrophils	0–4	0.00–0.36
Segmented neutrophils	50–70	2.00–6.30
Monocytes	2–8	0.08–0.72
Lymphocytes	25–45	1.00–4.05

Monocytes: the transitory precursors of the macrophages found in circulating blood.

Note: The occurrence of other leukocyte cell forms in a blood smear should be considered as abnormal and, therefore, pathologic.

3.4   Thrombopoiesis

3.4.1   Development of the Platelet-Forming Cell System in Bone Marrow

The morphologic process of thrombopoiesis is not comparable to that of erythropoiesis or granulopoiesis because the development of mature functional cells from immature precursors, with clear distinguishing morphologic characteristics and successive maturational divisions, does not take place. Instead, a polyploidization process occurs whereby successive duplication of DNA leads to the development of cells with 1 to 32 nuclei (2N to 64N), corresponding to different functional states. Rarely occurring endomitosis does not alter the principle of the polyploidization process. Three different cell types can be identified.

Megakaryoblast (Fig. 18a–d).   This cell generally is distinctly larger than proerythroblasts, with a high nuclear-to-cytoplasmic ratio. The nucleus is often tetraploid or octaploid, with variable chromatin density. Numerous, but mostly concealed, nucleoli with small centrospheres occur in the inner nuclear region. Although mononuclear cells predominate, cells with two to four nuclei also exist (products of rare endomitosis). The cytoplasm is strongly basophilic, free of granulation, and may be frayed at the edge. Sometimes, adhering platelets exist.

Promegakaryocyte (Semimature Megakaryocyte) (Fig. 18e–f).   Large, polyploid product of the megakaryoblast. Unlobed giant nuclei exist alongside forms that already have a clearly recognizable segmented (lobular) tendency. Nuclear chromatin predominates as a mesh, and nucleoli are mostly concealed. The cytoplasm is weakly basophilic, with discrete azurophilic granules that begin to show thrombopoietic activity. A distinct increase in the cytoplasmic width is apparent, and platelet adhesion occurs at the cell periphery.

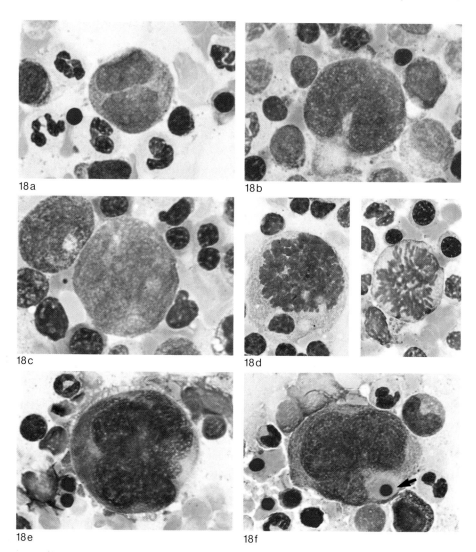

18a

18b

18c

18d

18e

18f

Fig. 18. Thrombopoiesis. **a–b,** Typical megakaryoblasts (bone marrow). **c,** Multinucleated megakaryoblast. **d,** Prophase nuclear changes in megakaryoblasts. **e–f,** Typical promegakaryocytes (bone marrow). **f,** Emperiopolesis of a normoblast (arrow) (a real diffusion or only a superimposition effect in the promegakaryocyte). Note: Observe the proportion of megakaryoblasts and megakaryocytes to the surrounding bone marrow cells.

Mature Megakaryocyte (Fig. 19a–b).   Under normal conditions, this cell is the largest hematopoietic cell in the bone marrow. This maturation product of the promegakaryocyte shows development of the typical nuclear shape and finely granulated azurophilic cytoplasm, which is the active expression of platelet formation. Occasionally, clusters of azurophilic cytoplasm microparticles are evident and correspond to preparation for platelet release. This course of events is observed particularly well with PAS staining (Fig. 19e–f). A few megakaryocytes (less than 10%) show, along with a decrease in diameter, small round to oval mononuclear or binuclear cells (so-called microkaryocytes), which also possess the thrombopoietic activity. Of particular note in the megakaryocyte is the migration of mature granulocytes through the cytoplasm without disturbing the cell integrity and without any indication of a phagocytic process (Fig. 19c–d).

Release of Platelets.   The cytoplasm of the active megakaryocytes breaks down with the formation of numerous microparticles having fine azurophilic granulation; these particles are the mature platelets. Cytoplasm-free residual nuclei remain detectable in the bone marrow until they are destroyed by macrophages, and caution must be taken against diagnostic error in scanning for carcinoma cells.

Platelet (Thrombocyte) (Fig. 20a–b).   This product of maturation of the cytoplasm of the megakaryocytes is released into the peripheral blood. The platelet is the smallest particle in the blood smear (about one-fourth to one-fifth the size of an erythrocyte), and consists of pale basophilic cytoplasm and azurophilic granulation. The physiologically spontaneous autoagglutination (aggregation) properties of platelets result in the close association of several platelets in smear specimens. Use of blood collected in EDTA is therefore recommended.

3.4.2   Basic Rules for Thrombopoiesis

Megakaryoblast: least mature cell form of thrombopoiesis, which develops into the promegakaryocyte by endoduplication of the nucleus.

Promegakaryocyte: product of a continuing polyploidization process that started in the megakaryoblast. Usually platelet formation does not yet occur.

Megakaryocyte: maturation product of promegakaryocytes. These are the true plateletforming elements of thrombopoiesis.

The true megakaryocyte content of a bone marrow aspirate can only be determined from perfect bone marrow smears.

Platelet: the only blood cell type that is exclusively a cytoplasmic maturation product.

All the cells of thrombopoiesis possess a cell-specific capacity for aggregation with platelets, which are therefore frequently found adhering to the edge of the cytoplasm of their mother cells. Similarly, platelets are found in aggregates, adhering to each other.

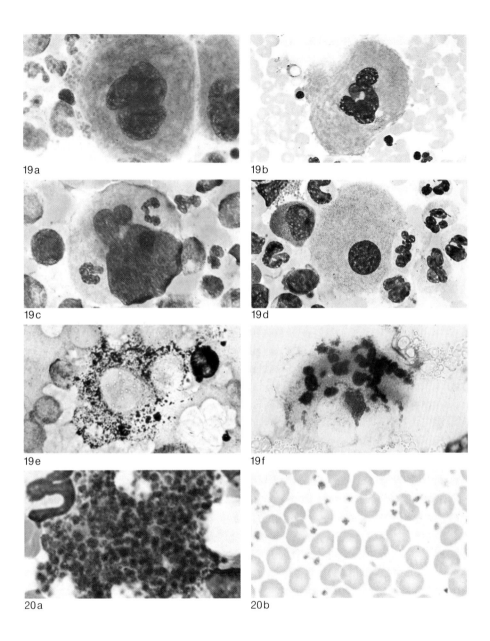

19a
19b
19c
19d
19e
19f
20a
20b

Fig. 19. Thrombopoiesis (bone marrow). **a–b,** Mature megakaryocyte with typical granulation in the cytoplasm. **c,** Emperipolesis of granulocytes in a megakaryocyte. **d,** Physiologic microkaryocyte (up to 10% of all megakaryocytes in normal bone marrow). **e,** Megakaryocyte at the stage of platelet discharge (PAS stain). **f,** Glycogen aggregate in megakaryocyte (sign of activity; PAS stain). Note the unstained nuclei in **e** and **f.**

Fig. 20. **a,** Platelet aggregate in blood smear. **b,** Single platelets in an EDTA blood smear.

3.5   Reticuloendothelial System (RES) (Reticulohistiocytic System [RHS]) and Monocyte-Macrophage System (MMS)

3.5.1   Elements of the RES and MMS in Bone Marrow

Stroma Cells.   The true reticulum cell and, at the same time, the structural cell of the bone marrow. The cells have a round- to oval-shaped nucleus, which contains a fine, loosely bound filamentous chromatin structure and pale blue nucleoli. The cytoplasm, because of its large size, is rarely seen in perfect condition in smear preparations, and even in relatively well-preserved cells, it is only recognizable on special staining for mesh fibers. Damage to the cytoplasm caused by the smearing technique leads to retraction and folding of the in vivo structure, which on silver staining (Gomori's) may be seen as a fine grid of reticulin fibers (Fig. 21a–b). On Wright's staining, these fibers sometimes produce an azurophilic tint. Occasionally, intracytoplasmic deposition of phagocytized material (cell fragments, stain, fat, or foreign bodies) may be seen. Isolated nuclei of the stroma cells are sometimes also described as "large reticulum cells."

Sinusoid Cell.   Also a true reticulum cell with an intracytoplasmic fibrous structure. The cells line the venous sinusoids of the bone marrow as typical vascular endothelia, and only rarely are seen in smear specimens as large elongated cell aggregates. The cells are seen mostly as isolated individual sinusoid cells with a round to oval nucleus that possesses the same chromatin structure and transparency as those of stroma cells. The nucleus, which has various shapes and is often elongated and blurred, is usually eccentrically situated in the cell and is encircled by the pale blue cytoplasm. In many of the cells, varying amounts of phagocytized material, mostly nuclear fragments and pigments, are found in the cytoplasm. In clusters of plasma cells (Fig. 21c), a centrally located reticulum cell, which corresponds to the sinusoid cell, may often be found. The sinusoid cells are a functionally important component of the monocyte-macrophage system in the bone marrow.

Macrophage.   The last cell of the monocyte-macrophage system, which is identical to the expression of the mononuclear phagocytic system (MPS). The macrophages, which are the tissue form of the blood monocyte, are formed from promonocytes in the bone marrow and circulate in the blood for only a short time before migrating to various organs, including the bone marrow. The macrophage is, therefore, the true functional form of the monocyte, whose primary functions are phagocytosis and pinocytosis (Fig. 21d–f), and is an important factor in the immunologic response of the organism.

A process can occur in which groups of erythroblasts extract ferritin molecules from the cytoplasm of macrophages by vesicle formation and subsequent incorporation (erythroblastic islands; Fig. 21g–h).

The morphology of the macrophage is often largely identical to that of individual sinusoid cells. Often seen are larger cells with various cytoplasmic inclusions (nuclear and cell fragments, pigments [see Fig. 21d], and degradation products of normal and pathologic metabolism, e.g., fat cells [see Figs. 21e–f; 67d–f]).

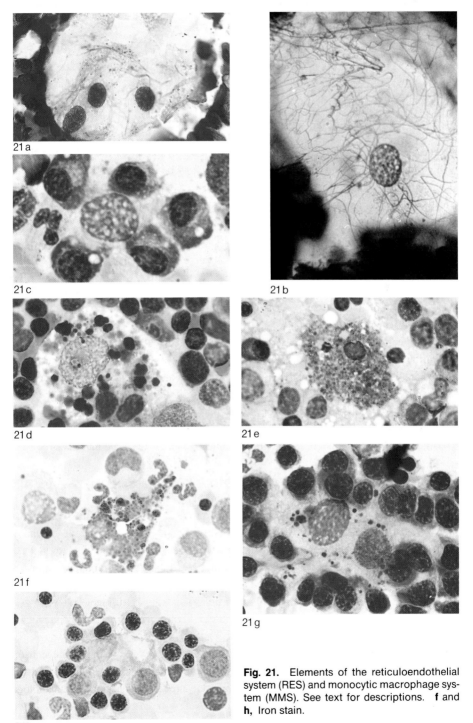

21a

21c

21b

21d

21e

21f

21g

21h

Fig. 21. Elements of the reticuloendothelial system (RES) and monocytic macrophage system (MMS). See text for descriptions. **f** and **h,** Iron stain.

Mast Cell (Tissue Basophil).   A cell form rarely seen in normal bone marrow smears; it is more pronounced in certain pathologic conditions. The nucleus is centrally located in the cells, and is round, violet (light or dark), and without characteristic structure. Often, the nucleus is nearly obscured by cytoplasmic granulation, and nucleoli are not clearly recognizable. The cytoplasm is round or polygonal, and is filled with small blue-black or violet-black granules, which, because of their extraordinarily tight packing, are barely recognizable individually. These granules often cover the cell nucleus and, when marrow smears are scanned, give the impression of a homogeneous black constituent. Granule-free mast cells, which are rarely found, have pink cytoplasm. Heparin, serotonin, and histamine are synthesized in mast cells.

Osteoblast and Osteoclast.   These cells, which mediate bone growth and degradation, are seen in bone marrow aspirates of adults only in rare pathologic conditions. Osteoblasts have a variety of shapes, but are mostly an elongated oval. They are characterized by a comparatively small, round- to oval-shaped and eccentrically situated nucleus, whose chromatin has a density similar to that of stroma cell chromatin. Small, light blue nucleoli can always be seen. The cytoplasm stains a pale blue, with a round gray-pink-tinted lighter area remote from the nucleus (archoplasm). Cytoplasmic granulation is absent. Osteoblasts are found in bone marrow aspirates in Paget's disease, in myelofibrosis with myeloid metaplasia, in metastatic osteoblastic carcinoma (e.g., in prostatic carcinoma), and less frequently in osteomalacia. Under normal physiologic conditions, osteoblasts are occasionally seen in marrow smears of children.

The osteoclast (Fig. 22a) is the largest cell observed in the bone marrow aspirate. It is a polyploid multinucleated (often containing 30 to 50 nuclei) giant cell. The nuclei are similar to those of the osteoblasts (Fig. 22c), with somewhat finer chromatin filaments. At least 1 nucleolus is seen in all cases. The cytoplasm is pale blue and always contains azurophilic granules. The granulation, in some instances, may be extremely dense, and thus, the blue of the cytoplasm may be obscured. Osteoclasts are found in bone marrow aspirates in osteitis fibrosa generalisata, osteomalacia, and metastatic osteoblastic carcinoma.

3.5.2   Basic Rules for the RES and MMS

The so-called reticuloendothelial elements of the human bone marrow originate predominantly from the blood monocytes; stroma cells and sinusoid cells are specifically recognizable as reticulum cells because of their reticulin fiber formation.

The tissue mast cells must be distinguished from blood basophils (Fig. 23b) (basophilic leukocytes), because the granulation of both types of cells is chemically identical (acid mucopolysaccharides).

Osteoblasts and osteoclasts do not belong to the reticuloendothelial system, and are included here for the sake of convenience as a rarely observed cell form.

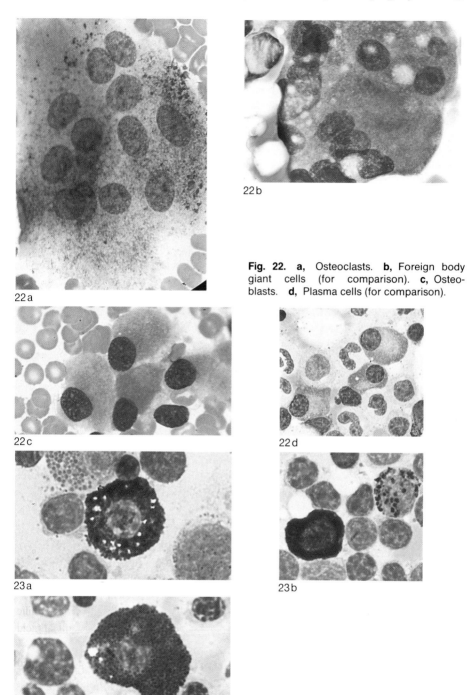

22a

22b

Fig. 22. a, Osteoclasts. **b,** Foreign body giant cells (for comparison). **c,** Osteoblasts. **d,** Plasma cells (for comparison).

22c

22d

23a

23b

23c

Fig. 23. Typical basophils (mast cells). **b,** A mast cell is alongside a blood basophil.

Single or crushed nuclei from different cells, as well as other artifacts, are often described as "reticulum cells." This error can only be avoided by careful preparation of the smear specimens and accurate observation of well-preserved cell elements.

A further differentiation of reticulum cells into dendritic forms depends on examination of the cells under the electron microscope using monoclonal antibodies.

3.6   Lymphopoiesis

3.6.1   The Cells of Lymphopoiesis (Fig. 24)

Lymphoblast (Reactive Lymphoblast Forms).   This is the stem cell of the small lymphocytes. The cell size varies widely and has a diameter that is sometimes larger than that of the blast cells in erythropoiesis and granulopoiesis. The cell shape is predominantly round, with a round nucleus showing a coarsely meshed, largely transparent chromatin structure that contains, in most cases, one or two blue or pale blue nucleoli. The cytoplasm is of varying width, lightly basophilic, and not granulated. The staining is deeper at the periphery and lighter centrally, and in some cases shows a perinuclear hyaloplasm zone. Under normal conditions, lymphoblast forms are not found in blood, but only in the lymph, where centroblasts and immunoblasts also appear (Fig. 25a–b). The term lymphoblast should be used only to describe pathologic conditions (see section 5.3.2).

Prolymphocyte.   This name is given to a cell form that is difficult to characterize and that morphologically lies between the large lymphoblast forms and the lymphocytes (Fig. 25a). This cell form, like the lymphoblast, is usually found only in the lymph. Also, prolymphocytes are reactive cell forms and not precursors of lymphocytes. Under pathologic conditions, prolymphocytes can be increased in the blood in chronic lymphatic leukemia or may appear in an independent leukemic disease (see Figs. 75a; 78).

Lymphocyte.   The differentiation of lymphocytes as "mature" and "immature" is no longer justified because several routes of lymphopoiesis have been recognized. The "mature" lymphocyte is thus an immature cell that, at all times, is capable of a blast transformation and is best classified only according to size. We therefore distinguish between the large and the small lymphocyte Fig. 26. Further morphologic subdivision according to origin and function is at present only partially valid. Possibilities for specific cytologic or cytochemical differentiation are shown in Figure 27. Consequently, the B-lymphocytes are more difficult to differentiate morphologically than are the T-lymphocytes. Only through the application of monoclonal antibody markers has an accurate identification of individual lymphocyte subpopulations become possible. The T-lymphocytes originate in the bone marrow and reach the thymus, thereby secondarily occupying certain regions of the lymphatic organs. The B-lymphocytes, on the other hand, go directly from the bone marrow to the lymph nodes, particularly to the germ centers. Additionally, specialized lymphocytes in the bone marrow possess stem cell properties for the entire hemopoietic process. The T-lymphocytes are responsible for the cellular and the B-lymphocytes for the humoral immune reaction (through transformation into plasma cells). The proportion of T-lymphocytes in the peripheral blood is 60 to 80%, and that of B-lymphocytes is 15 to 20%. The remaining lymphocytes,

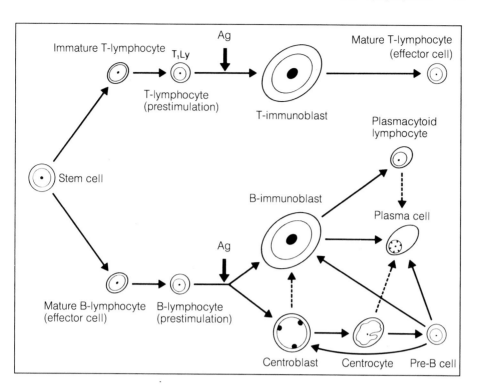

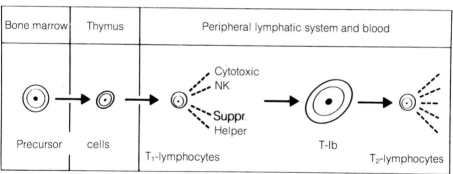

Fig. 24. a, Simplified schematic representation of lymphopoiesis. **b,** Simplified schematic representation of T cell development. Cytotoxic = cytotoxic cells; NK = natural killer cells; Suppressor = suppressor cells; Helper = helper cells; T-Ib = T-immunoblast.

a maximum of 10%, are called null cells and are the "natural killer (NK)" cells. Approximately two thirds of the T cells are helper cells; the remainder are suppressor cells or cytotoxic effector cells. The B_2- and T_2-lymphocytes (see Fig. 24) functional as so-called "memory cells" (elements of the immunologic memory).

Small Lymphocyte.   These cells are slightly larger than erythrocytes, and normally represent 95% of all lymphocytes in the peripheral blood. They possess a small basophilic cytoplasm, which occasionally appears to be discretely vacuolized. The nucleus is round or slightly kidney shaped, with a dense, coarsely lumpy, marbled chromatin structure. Nucleoli are occasionally seen without special staining as small bright points. In small lymphocytes with a somewhat wider cytoplasm, one occasionally can find coarse or fine azurophilic granulation that is indicative of suppressor cells. An increase in the cytoplasmic basophilia has led to the concept of the excited lymphatic form, which sometimes precedes the transformation into plasma cells (plasmablasts).

Large Lymphocyte.   This may be characterized first by an increase in the width of the cytoplasm. The cytoplasm is often a lighter blue than that of the small lymphocytes, and azurophilic granules may appear in larger numbers. The nucleus is more variable in shape and chromatin structure, and it is usually more transparent than that of the small lymphocyte. The so-called NK cells (see Fig. 26c) probably belong in this cell category (LGL, large granular lymphocytes). **Note:** An occasional spindle- or boat-shaped deformation of the lymphocytes (Fig. 27f) is probably an artifact and should be considered as such.

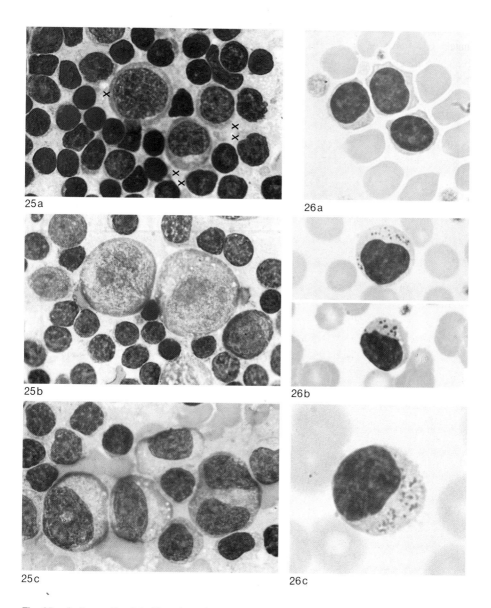

Fig. 25. Antigen-stimulated lymphopoiesis in lymphatic tissue (lymph node touch preparation, ×1000). **a,** Small lymphocytes, with one large and two smaller blasts (low degree of antigen stimulation); centroblast **(X)**, prolymphocytes **(XX)**. **b,** Strong blast transformation phase under intensive antigen contact with small lymphocytes, with two typical immunoblasts (center). **c,** Reactive lymphopoiesis with lymphoid cell characteristics of infectious mononucleosis (T-lymphocyte formation phase).

Fig. 26. Blood smear (buffy coat, ×1200). **a,** Small lymphocytes; difference between B and T cells not recognizable. **b,** Larger lymphocytes, with some azurophilic granulation, probably suppressor cells. **c,** Large lymphocyte with azurophilic granulation ("large granular lymphocyte," natural killer [NK] cell) **(×1500).**

3.6.2   Plasma Cells

When the discovery became known that plasma cells are formed from B-lymphocytes, plasma cells were reclassified into the lymphatic cell system. This lymphatic genesis through plasmablast precursors (Fig. 27c) (consisting of a centrally located nucleus containing dense chromatin and several nucleoli, and a narrow dark blue cytoplasm) can only be unequivocally proved morphologically in the lymphatic tissue. For bone marrow plasma cells (Fig. 28b–c), such formation has yet to be demonstrated. Both the plasmacytoid lymphocytes and those found in the bone marrow are capable of synthesizing immunoglobulins.

A basic morphologic differentiation between the two categories of plasma cells is rather difficult. Generally, if only the final cells are considered, the plasmacytoid lymphocytes are smaller, they tend to be less vacuolized, and their perinuclear bright zone is less pronounced (Fig. 27d). Most probably only the plasmacytoid lymphocytes reach the peripheral blood under reactive conditions.

Fig. 27. Significant cytochemical characteristics of lymphocytes on Wright's staining. **a,** Azurophilic granulated suppressor cell. **b,** Natural killer cell. **c,** Lymphatic plasmablast (B cell). **d,** Plasmacytoid lymphocyte. **e,** Lymphocyte with small satellite nucleus (chromosome defect?). **f,** Spindle lymphocyte. **g,** Lymphoid cell. **h,** Centrocyte. **i,** T-lymphocytes, with focal regions of positive acid phosphatase reaction. **k,** Lymphocytes with positive acid phosphatase granulation (found in B- and T-lymphocytes). **l,** T-lymphocytes with focal regions of positive esterase reaction. **m,** T-lymphocytes (helper cells) with positive diaminopeptidyl peptidase (DAP IV) reaction (see p. 117). **n,** Single T-lymphocyte with B-lymphocytes in chronic lymphocytic leukemia (CLL) (DAP IV reaction). **o,** The same smear as in **n,** stained with Wright's stain (arrow, helper cell). Note: Only in an almost exclusive B-lymphocyte population is it possible, with conventional staining techniques, to suspect T-lymphocytes, which appear as small cells with a densely chromatin nucleus.

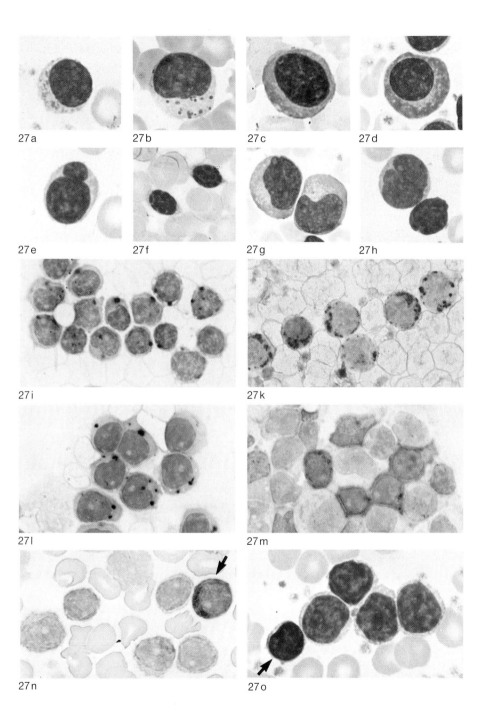

27a 27b 27c 27d

27e 27f 27g 27h

27i 27k

27l 27m

27n 27o

In the bone marrow smear, the plasma cells of marrow origin are seen as isolated cells or aggregated into small groups, often around a sinusoid cell (see Fig. 21c). The cell nucleus, which is usually eccentrically located, is circular and characterized by its pronounced coarse droplet-shaped chromatin structure. Between the individual chromatin particles are small lighter areas, which give the "cart wheel" appearance of the nucleus. Cell forms with two and more nuclei can occur (Fig. 28d). The cytoplasm is mostly pale blue, or in some cells somewhat darker blue (sky blue), with a wide and often irregularly shaped perinuclear bright zone. Vacuoles of varying number and size can often be seen in the cytoplasm. Under certain conditions, these vacuoles are filled with opalescent droplets (Russell bodies) (Fig. 28h), which correspond to solidified globulins. The appearance of the globular vacuoles ranges from single droplets to complete filling of the cell body, in which case the vacuoles may even obscure the nucleus. Following rupture of the cell membrane, the globular bodies may be seen dispersed between other marrow elements. In some plasma cells, the Russell bodies give a positive PAS reaction. In rare cases, one may find intracytoplasmic deposition of protein crystals, azurophilic plasma occlusions, or droplet-shaped bodies. Occasionally, plasma cells with a red-fringed cytoplasm are seen; these are called "flaming plasma cells." The function of these cells is not known, but they might contain high levels of IgA. A cytochemical change is observed in the degenerating plasma cell; the nuclear chromatin is maintained while the cytoplasm is considerably swollen and shows web-like structure.

3.6.3   Basic Rules for Lymphopoiesis

The term lymphoblast is limited to descriptions of acute leukemia. Blast forms that are
   detectable under physiologic conditions in lymph node preparations correspond to centroblasts or immunoblasts (see Fig. 25a–b).
Lymphocytes may be morphologically changed and disfigured to an exceptional degree
   during smear preparation and staining procedures.
Recent lymphocyte research has resulted in a departure from the rigid classification of the
   lymphocytes according to purely morphologic criteria. This change occurred because
   of the reliable proof of the capability of lymphocytes to change to blast forms in PHA
   (phytohemagglutinin or other mitogens) culture. Generally, all lymphatic cells in the
   peripheral blood are simply referred to as lymphocytes, and only special forms or features
   are given additional designations (e.g., azurogranulated, excited (stimulated) or reactive,
   or lymphoid forms).
T (thymus)- and B (bone marrow)-lymphocytes and their subpopulations, each having
   specific immunologic functions, can be only partially differentiated with special stains

Fig. 28. Plasma cells. a, Lymphatic plasmablast (precursor of blood plasma cell). **b–c,** Typical bone marrow plasma cells (under normal conditions, these have many variations). **d,** Double-nucleated bone marrow plasma cell. **e–g,** Protein occlusions in plasma cells. **g,** So-called Mott cell. **h,** Russell bodies (coagulated globulins) in plasma cells, with positive PAS reaction. **i,** So-called flaming plasma cell. **k,** Regressive changes in an atrophied plasma cell. Note: The plasma cell **(X)** in **c** is probably at the stage shortly preceding mitosis and represents the maximum size under normal conditions.

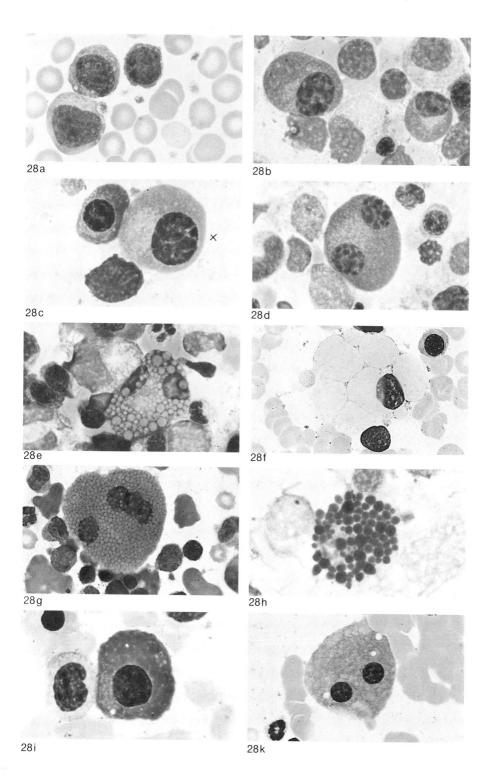

(acid phosphatase, acid esterase, DAP IV), but are reliably differentiated with mono-clonal antibodies (e.g., Leu 3a for helper cells, Leu 2a for suppressor/cytotoxic lym-phocytes).

Young children show a physiologic lymphocytosis in 50 to 70% of all leukocytes; this excess recedes slowly in the first decade. These juvenile lymphocytes do not show any mor-phologic peculiarities.

The number of lymphocytes in the total leukocyte content of peripheral blood is low under normal physiologic conditions. Lymphocyte values of 40 to 50% can occur transiently without any pathologic significance, but require monitoring. When the lymphocyte count falls below 20% ($<1000/\mu L$), an absolute lymphocytopenia is present if the granulocyte fraction of the differential blood count is normal or slightly elevated.

4 Morphologic Differential Diagnosis of the Most Important Cell Types and Cytochemistry of Normal Blood and Bone Marrow Cells

The only bone marrow and blood cells considered for comparison are those that are occasionally difficult to differentiate from each other.

Table 1.   Morphologic Differential Diagnosis of the Most Important Cells

Cell Type	Cell Shape	Nucleus	Nucleoli	Cytoplasm
Proerythro-blast	Round	Round; chromatin densely meshed, opaque	3 to 5, mostly obscured	Deep blue, with sickle-shaped perinuclear halo; no granules; characteristic earlets
Myeloblast	Nearly round	Bean shaped finely meshed, transparent	1 to 5, easily recognized by light blue color	Pale blue; narrower than in proerythroblast, with a less distinct perinuclear halo; no granules
"Lympho-blast" reactive lymphocyte	Nearly round	Round or indented; chromatin finely meshed, transparent	1 to 2, recognizable by pale blue color	Similar to myeloblast, but slightly broader; perinuclear halo in form of small droplets; no granules
Normoblast	Round	Round; centrally located, deeply colored chromatin, with distinct light- and dark-colored areas (clumping)	None	Narrow; nongranulated; may be basophilic, poly- or orthochromatophilic
Lymphocyte	Round to oval	Round or slightly indented; clumped chromatin, lighter color than in normoblast	1 to 4, mostly not visible	Narrow; half-moon shaped; light basophilic, lighter in fine droplets; may contain azurophilic granules
Plasma cell	Oval, egg shaped	Round; deeply stained, clumped chromatin with light areas, mostly eccentrically stratified	1, mostly not visible	Broad; irregular boundary, deeply basophilic; coarsely spotted perinuclear halo; may contain vacuoles; Russell bodies are specific, but rare

Table 1. (*continued*)

Cell Type	Cell Shape	Nucleus	Nucleoli	Cytoplasm
Promyelocyte	Round to oval	Round to oval, sometimes indented; chromatin finely meshed, moderately dense	2 to 3, often poorly visible	Medium to light basophils, lighter in area of nuclear indentation (centrosphere); contains azurophilic granules
Monocyte	Predominantly round	Indented (kidney shaped) or lobulated; chromatin coarsely meshed, transparent	1 to 2, usually not visible	Light basophilic, gray-blue color; fine azurophilic granulation
Myelocyte	Nearly round	Round or oval, slightly bean shaped, chromatin moderately dense; inhomogeneous	1 to 2, usually not visible	Pale gray-brown or pink, with fine violet granules; small light centrosphere
Metamyelocyte	Predominantly round	Bean shaped; chromatin dense, coarsely clumped, in distinct clusters	None	Similar to myelocyte; no centrosphere
Eosinophilic granulocyte	Round	Double segmented	None	Pale blue; often obscured by densely packed small round red or brown-red granules
Basophilic granulocyte	Round	Lobulated or multisegmented	None	Pink; contains widely distributed violet-black granules, mostly at cell perimeter and between nuclear lobes; vacuolated

4.1   Representative Pictures of Normal Bone Marrow

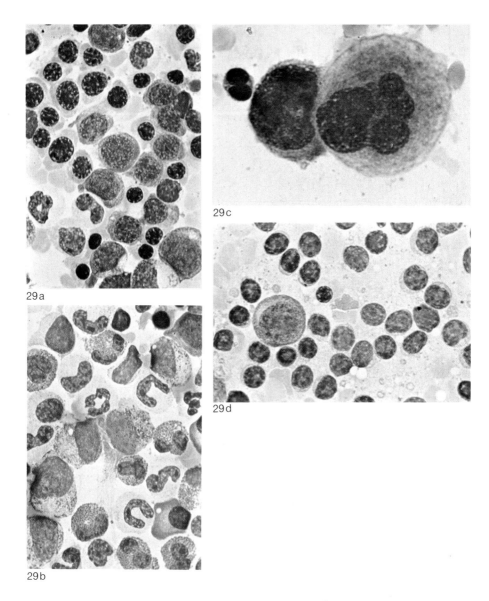

Fig. 29.   Normal bone marrow. **a,** Zone with erythropoietic activity[1] (× 1000). **b,** Normally maturing granulopoiesis[1] with eosinophils and plasma cells (× 1000). **c,** Megakaryoblast (left) and mature megakaryocyte (right) (× 1000). **d,** Section of lymph node from normal bone marrow (× 1000).

---

[1] Normally, the number of erythropoietic cells is 20 to 25% of the total, and that of granulopoietic cells is 60 to 70%, corresponding to an ME ratio of 3.0 to 3.5. The remaining 10% of cells consist of lymphocytes, plasma cells, and macrophages. Four to five megakaryocytes are usually found in every 1000 marrow cells. (These proportions were found by counting 1000 cells several times in technically perfect bone marrow aspirate preparations from healthy individuals.)

4.2 Cytochemistry of Normal Blood and Bone Marrow Cells

Table 2.   Cytochemistry of Normal Blood and Bone Marrow Cells*

Cell Type	Peroxidase	Nonspecific Esterase†	Periodic Acid– Schiff (PAS)	Acid Phosphatase	Comments
Myeloblast	− to (+)	(+)	− to diffusely (+)	−to (+)	
Promyelocyte	+ +	(+)	diffusely (+)	fine granules (+)	
Myelocyte	+ +	(+)	diffusely (+)	fine granules (+)	
Metamyelocyte	+ +	(+)	diffusely (+)	diffusely (+)	
Band neutrophil	+ +	(+)	+ to + +	diffusely (+)	Leukocyte alkaline phosphatase, grade 0–4, see below
Segmented neutrophil	+ +	(+)	+ +	diffusely (+)	
Eosinophil (granules)	+ +	−	− (cytoplasm +)	diffusely (+)	
Basophil (granules)	partly +	−	+ +	−	Metachromasia with toluidine blue
Monocyte (and precursors)	− to +	+ +	diffusely +	+ +	
Lymphocyte	−	focal partly (+) (acid esterase)	granules partly +	often + fine granules, and focal	T-lymphocytes DAP IV positive (see p. —)
Lymphocyte (reactive)	−	focal partly (+)	granules partly +	diffuse granules +	
Plasma cell	−	+	diffusely +	granules + +	Russell bodies; partly PAS positive
Proerythroblast	−	focal +	−	focal (+)	
Normablast	−	diffusely (+)	−	focal (+)	
Megakaryocyte (and precursors)	−	+	(+) to + +	+ +	
Platelet	−	+	+	+	
Macrophage	− to + to + +	+ +	+	+ +	Peroxidase positive, often contains phagocytic material
Tissue mast cell (granules)	(+)	−	+	−	Metachromasia with toluidine blue

* + +, Strong positive; +, positive; (+), weak positive; −, negative
† Inhibited by sodium fluoride.

Leukocyte alkaline phosphatase (see Fig. 63a–d)

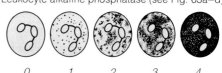

0   1   2   3   4

5   Morphology of Pathologic Changes in Blood and Bone Marrow

5.1   Morphologic Changes in Erythropoiesis in Disease

5.1.1   Basic Rules for Erythrocyte Morphology

Anisocytosis (variation in the size of erythrocytes) is a nonspecific morphologic change seen in all anemias. It is also found, to a small extent, under normal conditions.

Poikilocytosis (variation in the shape of erythrocytes) is an indication of a serious disturbance of erythropoiesis, of a hemoglobinopathy, of extramedullary erythropoiesis, or of peripheral mutilation of erythrocytes.

Poikilocytosis is mostly combined with an oval deformation of the erythrocytes, and thereby indicates an ineffective or aplastic erythropoiesis (panmyelopathy, pernicious anemia, myelodysplastic syndrome).

In contrast to the oval deformation of erythrocytes are the hypochromic anulocytosis (ring appearance resulting from deposition of hemoglobin around the cell periphery) of iron deficiency anemia and the microspherocytosis (spherical appearance) of hemolytic anemias.

A classification of most anemias is possible from careful observation of poikilocytosis, anulocytosis, and microspherocytosis. Also important for the classification of anemias is the reticulocyte count, especially as an indicator of the degree of activity of erythropoiesis in the bone marrow aspirate.

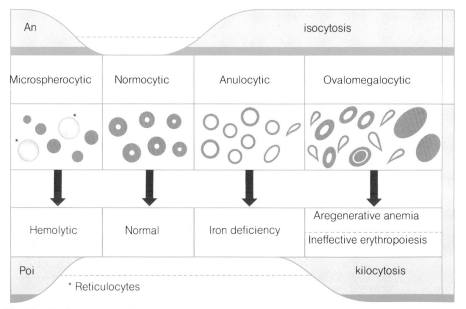

Fig. 30.   Erythrocyte morphology as a guide to the differential diagnosis of anemia.

5.1.2   Iron Deficiency Anemia

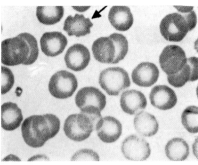

Fig. 31. Normal variation (mild anisocytosis) and central brightening (hemoglobin filling) of erythrocytes. Arrow shows crenated form—an artifact (Hb = 12.0 g/dl).

31

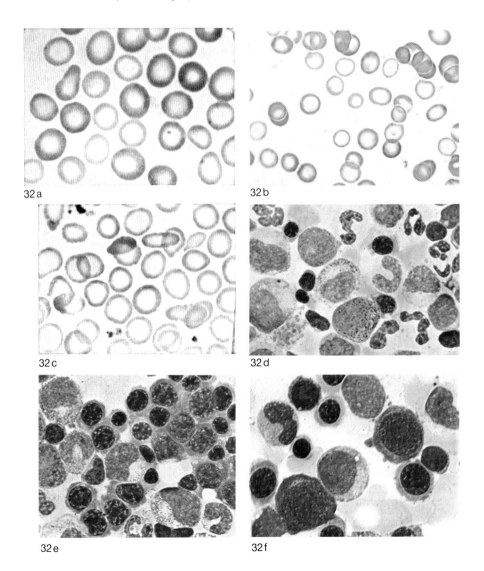

32 a

32 b

32 c

32 d

32 e

32 f

5.1.3   Pernicious Anemia

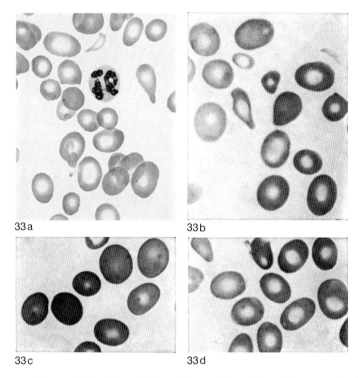

33a 33b

33c 33d

Fig. 33. Pernicious anemia. **a,** Typical blood picture shows ovalocytosis, anisomacrocytosis, and poikilocytosis of erythrocytes with hypersegmentation of granulocytes (×1000). **b–d,** Characteristic erythrocyte morphology in pernicious anemia: hyperchromia, oval macrocytosis (megalocytosis), and poikilocytosis (irregularly shaped erythrocytes, e.g., teardrop shaped, pear shaped, and dwarf forms). Note: Characteristic morphologic differences exist in comparison to iron deficiency.

Fig. 32. Iron deficiency anemia. **a,** Anisocytosis, moderate hypochromia (indicated by the ring form of the erythrocyte, also called anulocytosis). Anemia arising from chronic infection and many other origins. Typical erythrocyte picture of so-called secondary anemia. Note: Normochromia is seen in anemia from many infections. **b,** Marked anulocytosis and microcytosis (not always present) in chronic anemia caused by hemorrhage. **c,** Severe hypochromic microcytic anemia; essential iron deficiency anemia. There was no loss of blood, but there was a disturbance of iron resorption (from an 82-year-old female patient). **d,** Bone marrow in anemia caused by infection (erythropoiesis is not increased compared to granulopoiesis) (×800). **e,** Bone marrow in subacute hemorrhagic anemia: strongly regenerating erythropoiesis with cells at all stages of maturity (basophilic normoblasts). **f,** Bone marrow in true chronic iron deficiency anemia: slight stimulation of erythropoiesis, as in **e,** with strong regeneration (proerythroblasts +). Note: The so-called giant neutrophil bands, typical of pernicious anemia, are occasionally also seen in iron deficiency anemia.

5.1.4   Iron Storage in Bone Marrow

Cytochemical detection of stored iron (ferritin and hemosiderin) is obtained by a Prussian-blue reaction. Ferritin, at normal levels, cannot always be detected cytochemically, but in larger amounts, it produces a blue haze and streaks. Hemosiderin is found almost quantitatively in the form of granules and droplets. The stored iron is exclusively located in the cells of the reticuloendothelial system, such as macrophages or sinusoid endothelia, and for this reason is detected cytochemically in marrow smears that contain ample quantities of marrow particles. The amount of iron in the cell can be classified qualitatively (on a scale of 0 to 6+). Judgment of the classification of iron stores in the marrow requires training and experience and cannot be learned from descriptions in textbooks. Because the examination is made on fragments of aspirated marrow particles, care must be taken not to misinterpret the smears as false negatives. Removal of fat particles from the marrow smear preparation may be necessary to obtain a good stain (see p. 115).

Fig. 34. Iron storage in the bone marrow. **a,** Normal picture. **b,** Complete iron storage (true iron deficiency). **c,** A sideroblast with three siderosomes. **d,** Significantly increased iron storage (in moderate infection). **e,** Strongly increased iron storage (many causes: frequently found in severe infection, connective tissue diseases, and neoplasms without significant blood loss). **f,** Extreme iron storage (sideroblastosis, transfusion siderosis, hemachromatosis). **g,** Therapy: iron granules in sinusoids after iron therapy, either intravenous or with iron supplement (iron overload). (**a, b, d, e, f,** ×120; **c, g,** ×1000.) Note: The differential diagnosis of iron deficiency anemia (true iron deficiency or so-called anemia of infection) can be greatly facilitated by cytochemical observations of iron storage (compare **b** with **d** and **e**). The observation of sideroblasts (see **c**) in bone marrow aspirate confirms the diagnosis of a true iron deficiency or an extensive infectious anemia. The presence of sideroblasts with an increase in siderophilic granules is suggestive of ineffective erythropoiesis or hemolysis (sideroblastic anemia, see Fig. 41c). The observations in anemia caused by chronic renal disease are different.

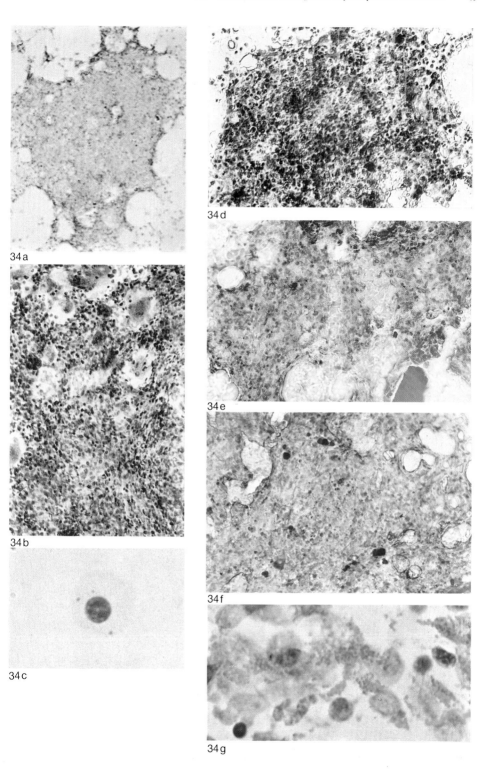

34a

34b

34c

34d

34e

34f

34g

5.1.5   Megaloblastic Erythropoiesis in Pernicious Anemia (Vitamin B₁₂ or Folate Deficiency)

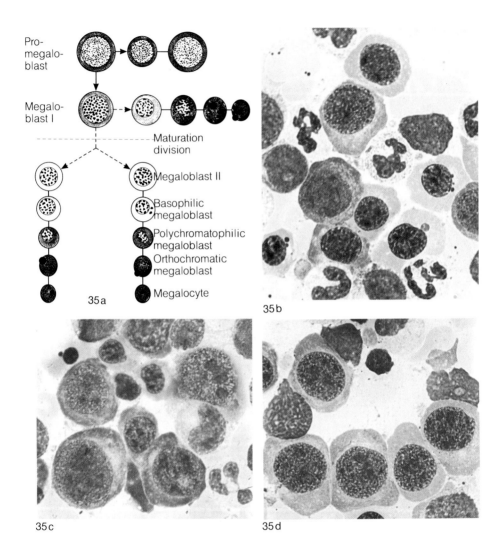

Fig. 35. Bone marrow in pernicious anemia.   **a,** Megaloblastic erythropoiesis; two maturation divisions do not take place because of a defect in DNA synthesis (for normal erythropoiesis, see pp. 10–14).   **b,** Megaloblasts at various stages of maturity alongside typical hypersegmented granulocytes.   **c,** Promegaloblasts, with typical cytoplasmic basophilia. Upper right, compressed promegaloblast with clearly visible nucleoli.   **d,** Polychromatic megaloblasts with typical nuclear-cytoplasm asynchronism and chromatin structure.

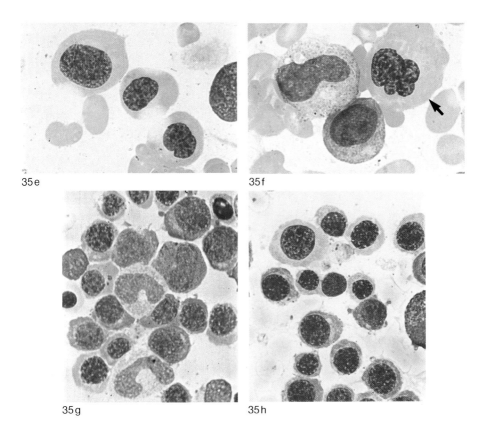

35e   35f

35g   35h

e, Mature megalonormoblasts.   f, Karyorrhexis (nuclear fragmentation) of a normoblast nucleus (arrow) (nuclear fragmentation results from inadequate cell division?).   g, Start of transformation of erythropoiesis under treatment with vitamin B_{12}; clear normoblastic tendency, during which giant neutrophilic bands persist for longer time periods.   h, Further maturation of erythropoiesis under specific therapy. (e and f are more highly magnified than g and h.) Note: In pernicious anemia, granulopoiesis is also affected (see Fig. 36).

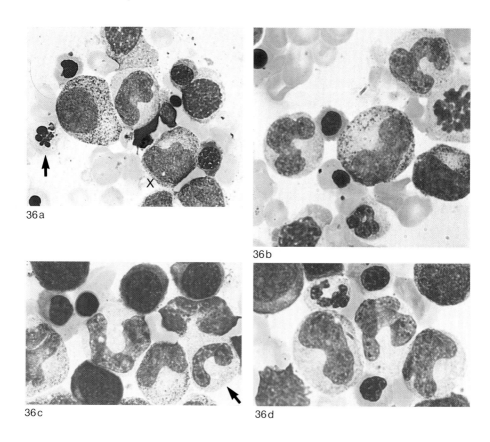

36 a

36 b

36 c

36 d

Fig. 36. Granulopoiesis and thrombopoiesis in megaloblastic anemia. a, Start of giant neutrophil band development; through the absence of maturation division the tendency for a transformation to giant neutrophil bands is recognizable even at the promyelocyte stage. The tendency for a transformation to giant neutrophil bands is recognized (X). Arrow shows karyorrhexis of a normoblast. **b,** A typical giant metamyelocyte between two giant neutrophil bands. **c,** Normal neutrophil band (arrow) alongside giant neutrophil band. **d,** Two giant metamyelocytes, one giant neutrophil band, and one hypersegmented granulocyte. **e,** Striking example of typical fine chromatin structure in a giant neutrophil band. **f,** Band form of a granulocyte with hypersegmentation **(arrow). g,** Megakaryocyte with typical hypersegmented nucleus. **h,** Extreme hypersegmented megakaryocyte (low magnification).

5.1.6   Granulopoiesis and Thrombopoiesis in Megaloblastic Anemia

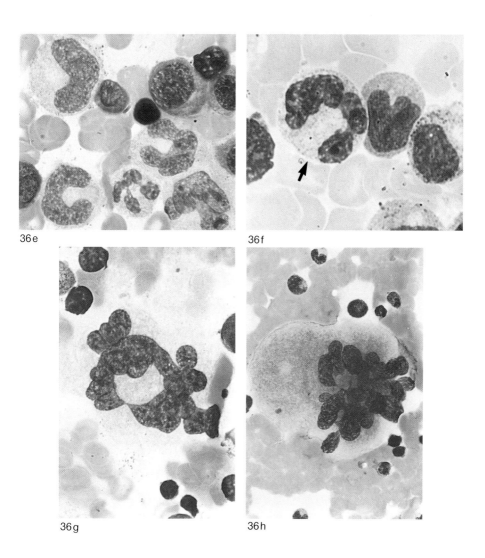

36e

36f

36g

36h

5.1.7   Hemolytic Anemia

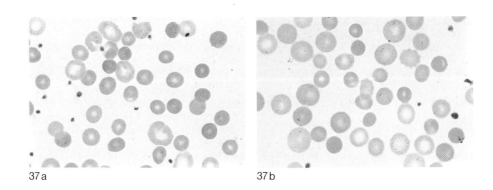

37 a   37 b

Fig. 37.   Hemolytic anemia (blood smear, × 800).
1. Erythrocyte-hereditary origin.   **a,** Hereditary spherocytosis (typical spherocytes).   **b,** Similar to **a,** but with evident polychromasia as an expression of a high reticulocyte count.   **c,** Hereditary stomatocytosis (rarely shows characteristics of hemolytic disease).   **d,** Acquired stomatocytosis in chronic alcoholism, for comparison with   **c.** Note: The additional oval macrocytic tendency of the erythrocytes results from concurrent existing folate and iron deficiency.
2. Autoimmune origin (acquired autoantibodies to erythrocytes detected by a positive direct or indirect Coombs' test).   **e,** Typical autoagglutination of erythrocytes in a blood smear. In this form of hemolysis, spherical cells can also appear.
3. Mechanical origin (hemolytic-uremic syndrome, effect of heart ventricle prosthesis, HELLP syndrome).   **f,** Typical distorted erythrocytes (poikilocytes, schistocytes) with a normoblast in the field.   Note: Echinocytes and acanthrocytes are erythrocytes with thorn-like or star-shaped protrusions that are found in uremia, pyruvate kinase deficiency, and disturbances in lipoprotein storage, and are visible as thorn-like forms in normal blood smears (artifact produced on drying and/or storing).
4. Toxic origin (chronic lead poisoning).   **g,** Clear basophilic stippling of erythrocytes as a consequence of a hemolytic change, a combination of toxic membrane damage and disturbance in hemoglobin synthesis as in lead poisoning.
5. Heinz body anemia.   **h,** Internally or peripherally located particle, generally attached to the erythrocyte membrane (only visible on supravital staining with crystal violet sulphate). Globulin precipitate found in denatured hemoglobin or in enzyme deficiency hemolytic anemias.   Note: Such disorders as paroxysmal nocturnal hemoglobinuria (PNH), which is associated with red cell membrane acetylcholinesterase deficiency, show no Heinz body deposition.
6. Bone marrow in hemolytic anemia.   **i,** Marked erythropoietic activity seen in all hemolytic anemias. As a consequence of the marked erythropoiesis there is a significant increase in the reticulocyte count. Arrow shows mitosis in a normoblast.   **k,** Hemolytic crisis (no regeneration in hereditary spherocytosis), with the formation of highly polyploid giant proerythroblasts and no reticulocytes.

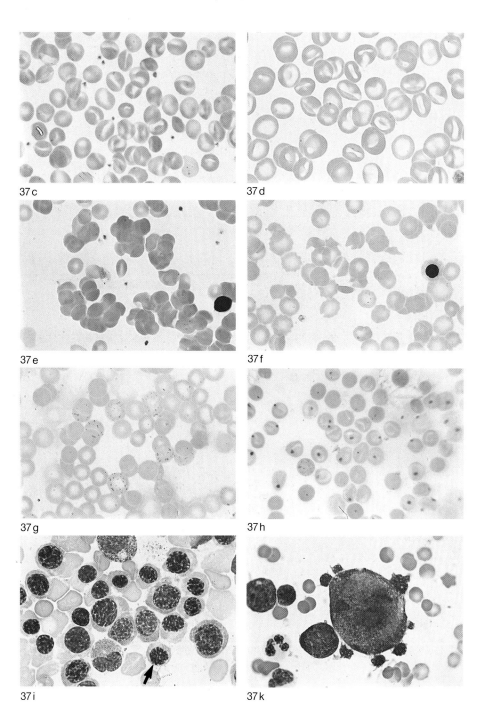

37 c

37 d

37 e

37 f

37 g

37 h

37 i

37 k

5.1.8   Advanced Hemolytic Syndrome

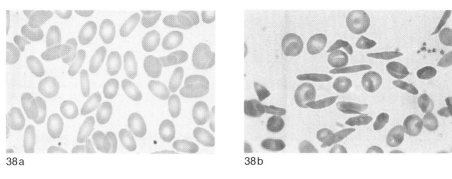

38a   38b

Fig. 38. a, Peripheral blood smear: ovalocytosis (elliptosis); a form of erythrocyte anomaly usually without anemia. **b,** Peripheral blood smear: sickle cell anemia (sometimes called drepanocytosis) from a patient with HbS disease.

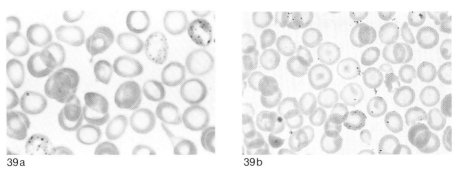

39a   39b

Fig. 39. Thalassemia (a case of heterozygous β-thalassemia). HbA$_2$ is usually increased, with or without an increase in HbF; sometimes called thalassemia minor. Peripheral blood smear: hypochromic erythrocytes (as in iron deficiency anemia), target cells, and basophilic stippling are usually present. Differential diagnosis from iron deficiency anemia: higher red cell count and plasma iron concentration. Note: In the homozygous form of β-thalassemia, numerous erythroblasts may be seen in the blood smear.

40

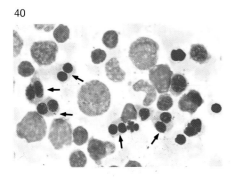

Fig. 40. Congenital dyserythropoietic anemia (CDA), type II (also known as hereditary erythroblastic anemia). Bone marrow ME ratio = 1. Significant double-nucleated normoblasts, along with karyorrhexis (×650). Note: The congenital dyserythropoietic anemias are rare autosomal recessive (types I and II) or autosomal dominant (type III) hereditary diseases of erythropoiesis.

5.2   Myelodysplastic Syndrome

With the introduction in 1982 of the FAB (French-American-British) classification of myelodysplastic syndromes, former names, such as hypercellular myopathy, preleukemia, and oligoblastic (or smoldering) leukemia, have been replaced by terms that better define the diseases. Some terms, however, such as sideroblastic and sideroachrestic anemias, have been retained under the FAB classification.

Five diseases of the myelodysplastic syndrome can be distinguished on the basis of hematologic criteria, although the boundaries are not always clear (Table 3).

Table 3.   Classification of Myelodysplastic Syndrome

Disease	Abbreviation	Bone Marrow	Peripheral Blood
Refractory anemia	RA	Ring sideroblasts <15%* Blasts <5%†	Blasts <5%
Refractory anemia with ring sideroblasts (formerly sideroachrastic anemia)	RARS	Ring sideroblasts >15% Blasts <5%	Blasts <5%
Refractory anemia with excess blasts	RAEB	Blasts 15–20%	Blasts <5%
Refractory anemia in transformation	t-RAEB	Blasts 20–30%	Blasts ≤5%
Chronic myelomonocytic leukemia	CMML	Blasts <20%	Monocytes ≤1 × 10^9/L

* % of nucleated erythropoietic cells
† % of nucleated marrow cells

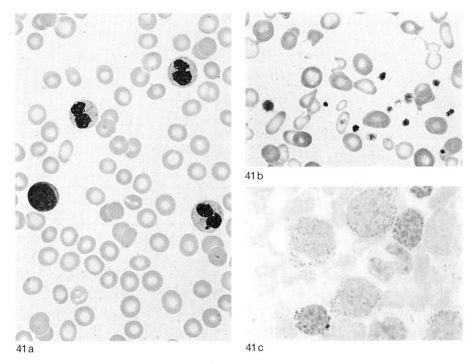

41 b

41 a   41 c

Fig. 41. Myelodysplastic syndrome.   a, Peripheral blood smear (low magnification): RAEB. Three granulocytes with Pelger-Huët nuclear anomaly next to a blast cell.   **b,** Peripheral blood smear: advanced RA with marked erythrocyte changes (oval anisocytosis and poikilocytosis).   **c,** Bone marrow (iron stain): RARS with numerous typical ring sideroblasts.   Note: See Table 3 for explanation of abbreviations.

Fig. 42. Myelodysplastic syndrome.   **a–b,** Bone marrow: megaloblastoid dyserythropoiesis, several sizes common to all myelodysplasias.   **c–d,** Bone marrow (low magnification): typical dysmegarkaryocytosis with mono- and binucleated cells predominating.   **e,** Bone marrow (t-RAEB): two blasts (arrow) in dyserythropoietic area.   **f,** Bone marrow: RAEB with dysgranulo-poiesis; promyelocyte with slight cytoplasmic basophilia (upper right), a type I myeloblast (bottom) beside (on the left) two megaloblastoid erythroblasts.   Note: See Figure 60b, p. 72, for a typical blood smear in CMML. See Table 3 for explanation of abbreviations.

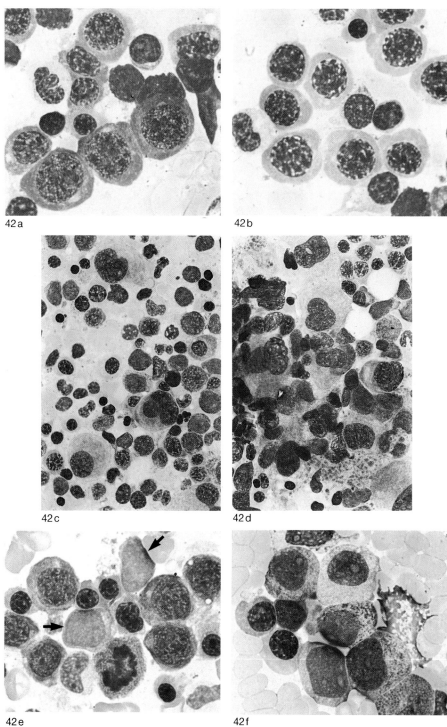

42a

42b

42c

42d

42e

42f

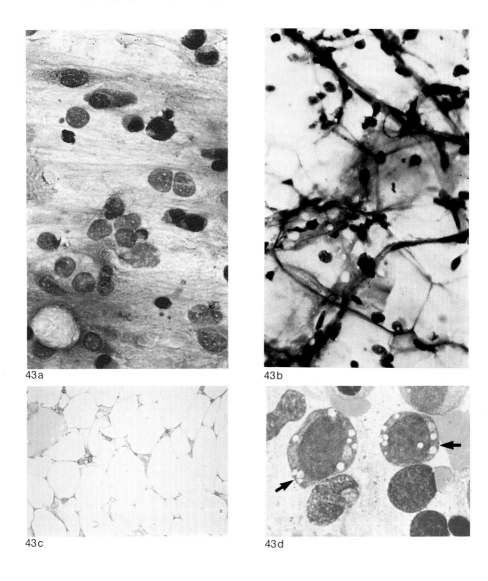

43a

43b

43c

43d

Fig. 43.   Aplastic anemia; panmyelopathy.   **a,** Bone marrow: widespread absence of hemato-poiesis; increase in fibroblasts and fat cells with few lymphocytes, reticulum cells, plasma cells, or tissue mast cells. Definitive diagnosis is made through bone marrow biopsy (hematoxylin and eosin) (see **c**).   **b,** Pure fibrotic marrow in sternal aspirate (found following x-ray irradiation of breast carcinoma as localized areas of disappearance of blood-forming tissue; × 400).   **d,** Vacuolized proerythroblasts (arrows) in bone marrow aspirate in toxic chloram-phenicol damage (early symptoms). Also seen in chronic alcoholism.

5.3 Morphologic Changes in Granulopoiesis in Disease

5.3.1 Hereditary and Reactive Changes

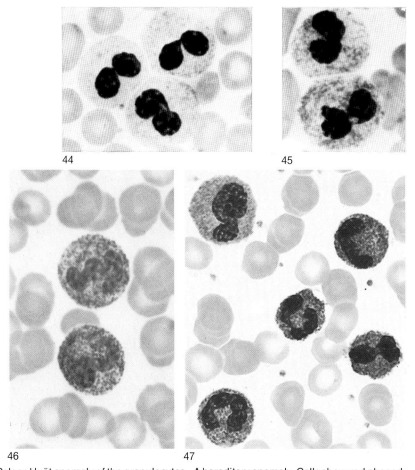

44   45

46   47

Fig. 44. Pelger-Huët anomaly of the granulocytes. A hereditary anomaly. Cells show rod-shaped or predominantly bisegmented nuclei; nuclear chromatin is noticeably coarse and lumpy, stimulating shift to the left.

Fig. 45. Pseudo-Pelger cells. Toxic reactive Pelger-Huët-like transformation of the granulocyte nucleus; chromatin structure less coarse and lumpy, cytoplasm mostly toxic, granulated. Occurs in toxic intestinal disorders, and possibly in chronic myelocytic leukemia or myelodysplastic syndrome. Reversion of the Pelger-like changes is possible, in contrast to the true Pelger-Huët anomaly.

Fig. 46. Alder-Reilly granulation anomaly of granulocytes, eosinophils, and basophils. Extreme azurophilic granulation, often obscuring a somewhat weakly stained nucleus. Hereditary anomaly, mostly in conjunction with mucopolysaccharidoses (gargoylism, Hurler's syndrome). Differential diagnosis includes the rarely seen Chédiak-Higashi-Steinbrinck syndrome, which has cytoplasmic granulation in all the leukocyte cell forms.

Fig. 47. Toxic granulation of granulocytes. Shows an increase in azurophilic granulation, but not as intensive as in the Alder-Reilly anomaly (Fig. 46). Good staining of the nucleus indicates that the cells were not overstained.

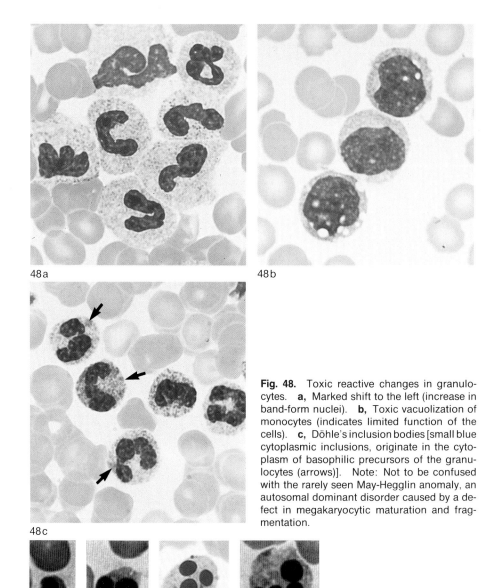

48a

48b

48c

Fig. 48. Toxic reactive changes in granulocytes. **a,** Marked shift to the left (increase in band-form nuclei). **b,** Toxic vacuolization of monocytes (indicates limited function of the cells). **c,** Döhle's inclusion bodies [small blue cytoplasmic inclusions, originate in the cytoplasm of basophilic precursors of the granulocytes (arrows)]. Note: Not to be confused with the rarely seen May-Hegglin anomaly, an autosomal dominant disorder caused by a defect in megakaryocytic maturation and fragmentation.

49a   49b   49c   49d

Fig. 49. Degradation forms of granulocytes. These occur rarely in vivo; confusion with normoblasts is possible. Often found in discharges from body cavities and in vitro (e.g., blood collected in EDTA and allowed to stand for 8 hours or longer).

Fig. 50. Eosinophilia of the blood (seen in allergies, parasitic infestation, Hodgkin's disease, and periarteritis nodosa). Note: Eosinophilic leukemia (a rare disease) shows peripherally immature eosinophilic cell forms.

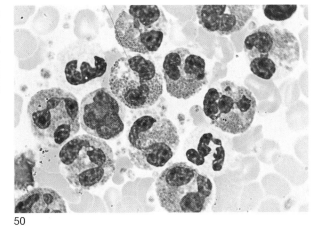

50

Fig. 51. LE cells (a phenomenon of systemic lupus erythematosus). **a,** Altered (homogeneous red-violet) nuclear material is phagocytized by a group of intact leukocytes (rosette formation). **b,** Single LE cell with phagocytized occlusion of a particularly large homogeneous and spherical nuclear mass; the nucleus lies on the edge of the cell.

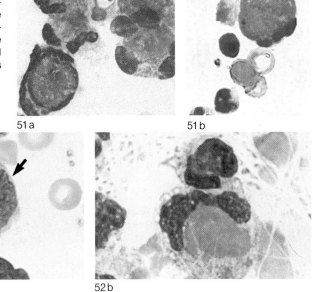

51a   51b

52a   52b

Fig. 52. Tart cell. **a,** Lymphophagocytosis of a monocyte (arrow) (nonspecific phenomenon). **b,** Pseudo-LE cell (joint fluid); monocyte phagocytosis leading to deposition of mucosulphates.

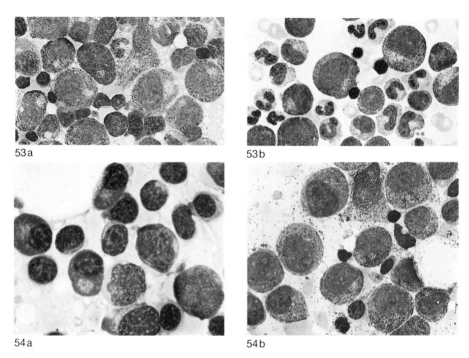

53a   53b

54a   54b

Fig. 53. Different functional states of granulopoiesis in the bone marrow. **a,** Shift to the left; the majority of the cells are promyelocytes and myelocytes. **b,** Shift to the right; the majority of the cells are metamyelocytes, and band and segmented neutrophils. Note: These phenomena are temporary changes in the normal mechanism of granulopoiesis; a shift to the left can be balanced by a shift to the right, but can also persist. The actual value of the peripheral granulocytosis is based on clinical information.

Fig. 54. Agranulocytosis. **a,** Bone marrow: so-called "empty marrow," marked granulocytopenia. Lymphocytes and plasma cells are present, along with megakaryocytes and areas of erythropoiesis. **b,** Bone marrow: so-called "full marrow" (promyelocytic marrow). Usually has a better prognosis than does "empty marrow." Single lymphocytes are between the promyelocytes. As a rule, the eosinophil line is maintained in agranulocytosis. Note: Remission of agranulocytosis gives the marrow picture shown in Figure 53b; in the peripheral blood, there is often no granulocytosis in spite of a "full marrow."

Definition of Leukemoid Reaction.   Appearance of immature precursors of erythropoiesis and granulopoiesis, rarely thrombopoiesis, in the peripheral blood. Origins: (1) excessive regeneration of an individual blood-forming system (e.g., remission stage of agranulocytosis [see Fig. 53b]; severe hemolytic crisis); (2) change in the bone marrow (e.g., myelofibrosis [see Fig. 62a]; bone marrow carcinoma [see Fig. 89]).

Footnote: Chronic leukopenia occurs, e.g., in hypersplenism (increase in the sequestration activity of the spleen in splenomegalic diseases, e.g., Felty's syndrome, splenic vein thrombosis). In the bone marrow, a compensatory granulopoiesis (mostly left shift) occurs, with eventual increase in erythropoiesis and thrombopoiesis, but without atypical cells.

5.3.2   Acute Leukemias (AL) and Myeloproliferative Diseases

Table 4.   FAB Classification of Acute Leukemias
(1976/1985: Myeloid Leukemias)

Abbreviation	Morphologic Characteristics	Type
M_1	Undifferentiated myeloblasts (type I)	AML I
M_2	Myeloblasts with early differentiation (Type II)	AML II
M_3	Promyelocytes with heavy granulation, multiple Auer bodies present	AML III
M_3 (var)	Variant with less granulation, bi- or multilobular nuclei, and few Auer bodies	AML III (var)
M_4	Immature granulopoiesis and monocytopoiesis with >30% myelomonoblasts	AMML
M_4–E_o	M_4 with abnormal eosinophils	AMML–E_o
M_5	Differentiated and undifferentiated monoblasts present	AMoL
M_6	Abnormal erythropoietic cells and myeloblasts present	AEL
M_7	Predominantly small megakaryoblasts present (rare)	AMegL

Abbreviations

AML I } AML II }	acute myeloblastic leukemia	AMML–E_o	acute myelomonocytic leukemia with abnormal eosinophils
AML III	acute promyelocytic leukemia	AMoL	acute monoblastic-monocytic leukemia
AML III (var)	variant of acute promyelocytic leukemia	AEL	acute erythroleukemia
AMML	acute myelomonocytic leukemia	AMegL	acute megakaryoblastic leukemia

Table 5.   Cytochemical Classification of Acute Myelocytic
Leukemias (Löffler)

Leukemia	Peroxidase	Esterase*	PAS†
AML I	} 1–64%	<10% (+)	−
AML II		<25% (+)	− to weak diffuse or fine granular +
AML III	>65% + +	<25% (+)	Like AML II, rarely granulated
AMML	Mostly <50% +	25–50% +	Diffuse − fine granular +
AMoL	<20% +	>50% + +	Sometimes fine granular +
AEL	−	Diffuse (+) and focal point +	Immature erythroblasts, granular +; mature forms, diffusely +

− negative, (+) weak positive, + positive, + + strong positive reactions.
* Nonspecific esterase (inhibited by sodium fluoride).
† Periodic acid–Schiff reaction.

Table 6.   FAB Classification of Acute Leukemia (1976):
Lymphoblastic Leukemias (ALL)

Abbreviation	Morphologic Characteristics	Lymphoblastic Type
L_1	Small cell	ALL/AUL
L_2	Mixed (some larger) cells	ALL/AUL
L_3	Burkitt-type, large cells, cytoplasmic vacuoles	ALL

AUL = acute undifferentiated leukemia; ALL = acute lymphoblastic leukemia.

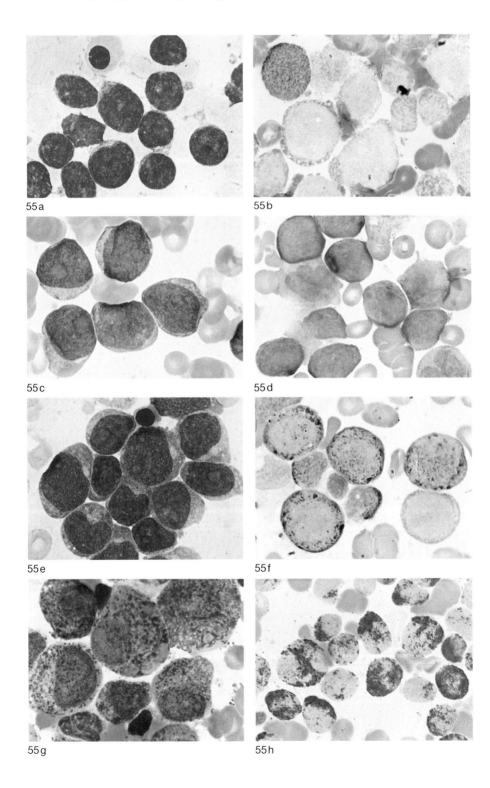

55a

55b

55c

55d

55e

55f

55g

55h

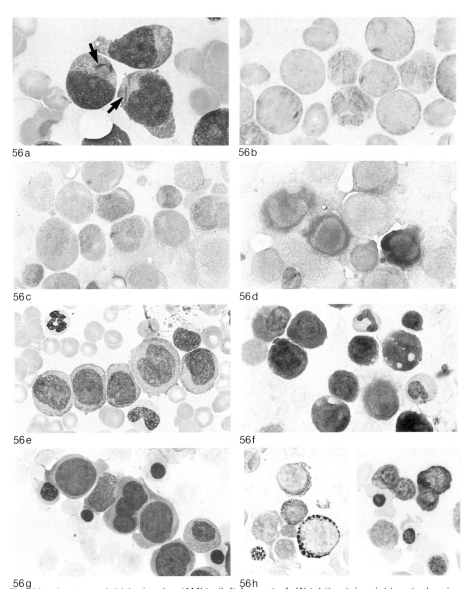

56a

56b

56c

56d

56e

56f

56g

56h

Fig. 56. Acute myeloid leukemias (AML); (left [except **c**], Wright's stain; right, cytochemistry). **a,** Acute myeloid leukemia (AML–M₂/AML–M₃) with Auer rods (arrows). **b,** Auer rods, peroxidase positive. **c,** Acute myelomonocytic leukemia (AMML) (M₄), a peroxidase-positive reaction. **d,** AMML (M₄), nonspecific esterase. **e,** Acute monocytic leukemia (AMOL) (M₅). **f,** AMOL (M₅), nonspecific esterase. **g,** Acute erythroleukemia (AEL) (Di Guglielmo disease). **h,** AEL (M₆), PAS-positive (granular in proerythroblasts, diffuse in normoblasts). **i,** Acute megakaryoblast leukemia (M₇) (bone marrow, Wright's stain). Note: PAS-positive erythroblasts are also found in ring sideroblasts, in thalassemia, and occasionally in iron deficiency.

Fig. 55. Acute myeloid leukemias (AML); (left, Wright's stain; right, cytochemistry). **a,** Acute undifferentiated (stem cell) leukemia. AML (M₁). **b,** Peroxidase negative upper left; a positive granulocyte. **c,** Acute myeloblastic leukemia (AML–M₁). **d,** AML–M₁, peroxidase weakly positive. **e,** Acute myeloblastic leukemia (AML–M₂). **f,** AML–M₂, peroxidase distinctly positive. **g,** Hypergranular promyelocytic leukemia (AML–M₃). **h,** AML–M₃, peroxidase strongly positive (×800). (Figures **g** and **h** courtesy of Prof. Löffler, Kiel.) (Schäfer and Fischer peroxidase reaction, see p. 113.)

Table 7.   Cytochemical Classification of Acute Lymphoblastic Leukemias (ALL)

Leukemia*	PAS†	AP‡	TdT§
c-ALL	>70% coarse, lumpy granular + +	−, rare cases (+)	+
T-ALL (L$_1$, L$_2$)	<40%, granular +	>80% focal + +	+
B-ALL (L$_3$)	− to (+)	granular (+)	−
B-ALL (AUL-lymphocytic origin)	− to (+)	− to (+)	+

− negative, (+) weak positive, + positive, + + strongly positive reactions.
* c-ALL, common acute lymphoblastic leukemia; T-ALL, T cell acute lymphoblastic leukemia; B-All, B cell acute lymphoblastic leukemia.
† Periodic acid–Schiff reaction.
‡ Acid phosphatase reaction.
§ Terminal deoxynucleotidyl transferase reaction.
Note: Further subtyping of ALL is only possible using monoclonal antibodies.

Table 8.   Examples of the Use of Monoclonal Antibodies for Hematologic Diagnosis

Monoclonal Antibody	Cell Type
To 15	Pan-B cell
Okt 10	Immature thymocyte (pre-T-ALL)
Okt 11, Leu 1	T-ALL, T-NHL
Okt 8, Leu 2a	T suppressor cell
Okt 4, Leu 3a	T helper cell

Note: A detailed list of monoclonal antibodies in current use is given in Table 12.

Fig. 57. Acute lymphoblastic leukemia (ALL) (left, Wright's stain; right, cytochemistry).   **a,** Common acute lymphoblastic leukemia (c-ALL) (L$_1$), arrows showing so-called hand-mirror form (also seen, rarely, in AML).   **b,** c-ALL (L$_1$), PAS-positive (+).   **c,** c-ALL (L$_2$).   **d,** c-ALL (L$_2$), PAS-positive (+ +).   **e,** T cell acute lymphoblastic leukemia (T-ALL).   **f,** T-ALL, acid phosphatase-positive (+ +) spots.   **g,** B cell acute lymphoblastic leukemia (B-ALL) (Burkitt).   **h,** T-ALL, fluid sediment in meningiosis, acid phosphatase-positive (+).

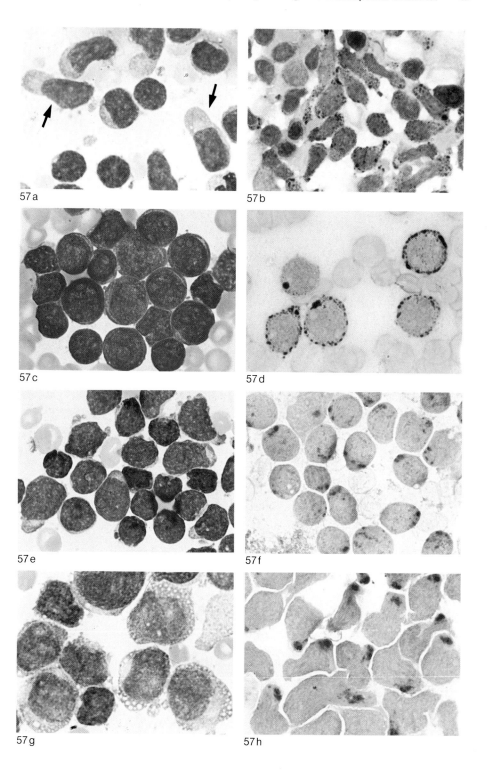

57 a

57 b

57 c

57 d

57 e

57 f

57 g

57 h

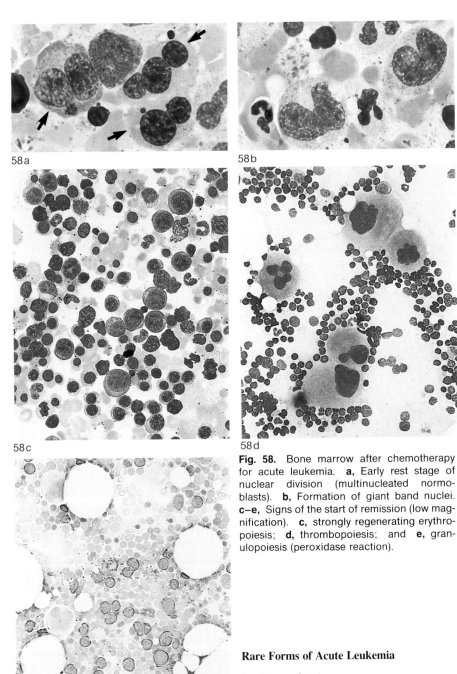

58a

58b

58c

58d

Fig. 58. Bone marrow after chemotherapy for acute leukemia. **a,** Early rest stage of nuclear division (multinucleated normoblasts). **b,** Formation of giant band nuclei. **c–e,** Signs of the start of remission (low magnification). **c,** strongly regenerating erythropoiesis; **d,** thrombopoiesis; and **e,** granulopoiesis (peroxidase reaction).

Rare Forms of Acute Leukemia

(no illustrations)

1. Neutrophilic leukemia.
2. Eosinophilic leukemia.
3. Basophilic leukemia.

58e

Table 9.   Myeloproliferative Disease

Disease	Peripheral Blood Smear*	Bone Marrow*	ALP Index†
Chronic myelocytic leukemia (CML) Stage 1 (early stage)	Leukocyte count: <50 × 10⁹/L; single immature cells, basophils eventually (+).	Very cellular. ME‡ ratio 5–6. Granulopoiesis significantly shifted to the left. Increase in number of basophils and eosinophils. Mega- and microkaryocytes (+).	<10
Stage 2 (complete picture)	Leukocyte count: 50–500 × 10⁹/L. All cell forms of granulopoiesis present. Fraction of blasts relative to total cell count <5%, (small) basophils +, platelet count often >400 × 10⁹/L.	Extremely cellular, no fat cells, ME ratio > 10. Granulopoiesis with distinct left shift, but sufficient maturation. Basophils, eosinophils, and microkaryocytes + +. Gaucher's cells rarely present and blasts not present.	<10, mostly 0
Stage 2–3 (accelerating phase)	Leukocyte count: up to 250 × 10⁹/L; immature forms + + (promyelocytes 20–30%), blasts up to 10%, basophils + +, platelet count normal.	Similar to stage 2, with strong left shift and a significant increase in promyelocytes. Proportion of blasts ~10%.	0–5
Stage 3 (blast phase)	Blasts: mostly >5%, almost 100% in the final stage (25% TdT- or PAS-positive). The other cell types as in stage 2 with some atypia. Thrombocytopenia +.	Blastic marrow with significant numbers of mature granulopoietic cells. Immature basophils +. Reduced erythropoiesis and thrombopoiesis. PAS-positive blasts in ~25% of stage 3 cases.	0–150
Chronic megakaryocytic (granulocytic) myelosis (CM(G)M)	Leukocyte count: max. 50 × 10⁹/L; significant number of immature leukocytes, thrombocytosis often present; final blastic step or transformation to myelofibrosis.	Cellular, but difficult to aspirate because of premature fiber development. ME ratio ~5. Granulopoiesis shifted significantly to the left. Megakaryocytes + + +, with many cells having bizarre nuclei.	>100
Polycythemia vera (p.v.)	Erythrocyte count elevated, leukocyte count: 10–30 × 10⁹/L; granulocytes +; rare left shift, often toxic granulation. Platelet count 150–450 × 10⁹/L. Transformation to OMF.	Stimulation of all three types of blood cells, development (panmyelosis), with changes in the fat cells. Megakaryocyte nuclei often lobulated. Stored iron mostly negative.	150–400
Osteomyelofibrosis (OMF)	Poikilocytosis of erythrocytes +; leukocyte count: 10–100 × 10⁹/L; typical leukemoid reaction with blasts, pro- and myelocytes, erythroblasts. Platelet count normally increased, macrothrombocytes and megakaryocyte nuclear fragments often present.	Marrow cells are only seen in the early stages of the disease. Marrow rich in megakaryocytes with bizarre nuclei. Otherwise normal features. Histologic marrow staining is required.	0/<100/>100
Idiopathic thrombocytopenia purpura (ITP)	Erythrocyte and leukocyte counts normal. White cell differential unremarkable. Platelet count 0.6–2.0 × 10¹²/L; macrothrombocytes + (**Note:** megakaryocytic myelosis.)	Cellular, but fat cells predominate. Essentially normal erythropoiesis and granulopoiesis. Significant increase in number of large megakaryocytes with bizarre nuclei.	Normal

(+), +, + +, + + +: scale indicating presence of cells.
* Abbreviations used: TdT, terminal deoxynucleotidyl transferase reaction; PAS, periodic acid–Schiff reaction.
† ALP index: for classification using leukocyte alkaline phosphatase, see p. 111.
‡ ME ratio: quantitative comparison of granulopoiesis and erythropoiesis (see pp. 42, 104–105)

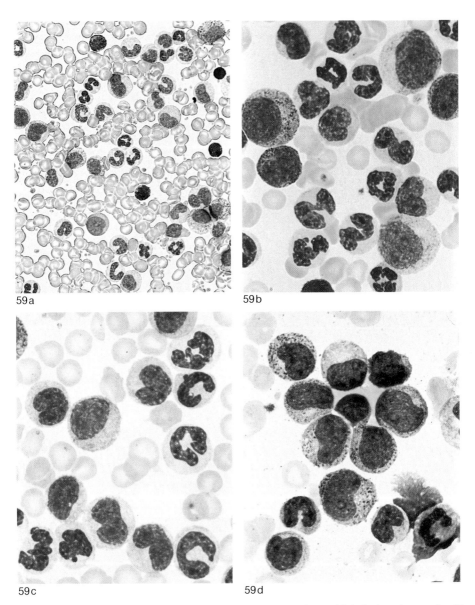

Fig. 59. Chronic myelocytic leukemia (CML) (blood smear). **a,** High leukocyte count, with increase in left shift to the blasts (typical stage 2 picture) (overview, ×250). **b,** Enlargement of **a** (×1200). **c,** Stage I few immature cells in the differential blood picture. **d,** Stage II–III, accelerating disease stage, with >20% promyelocytes.

Fig. 60. Chronic myelocytic leukemia (blood smear). **a,** Stage II, increased formation of eosinophils (arrows). **b,** Chronic monocytic form (rare). **c,** Typical increase in basophils (stage II). **d,** Malignant basophil (stage III). **e,** Same as **d,** with toluidine blue stain. **f,** Blast (stage III). **g,** Other blast forms in stage III. **h,** Lymphoid blast (PAS reaction, partly positive granules).

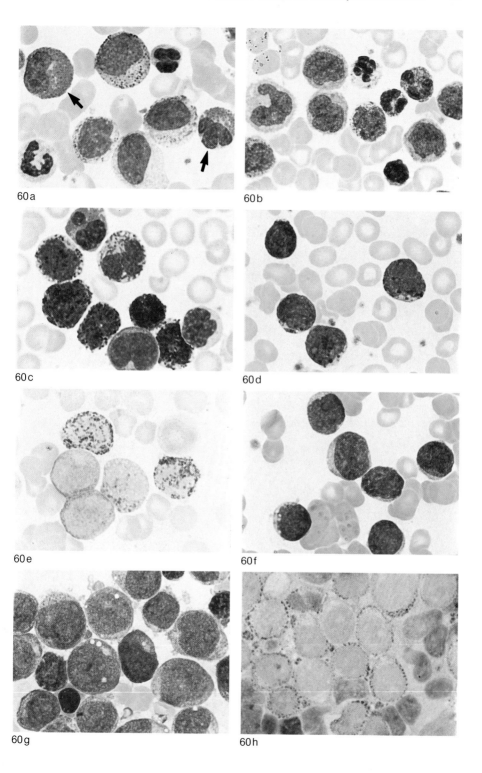

60a

60b

60c

60d

60e

60f

60g

60h

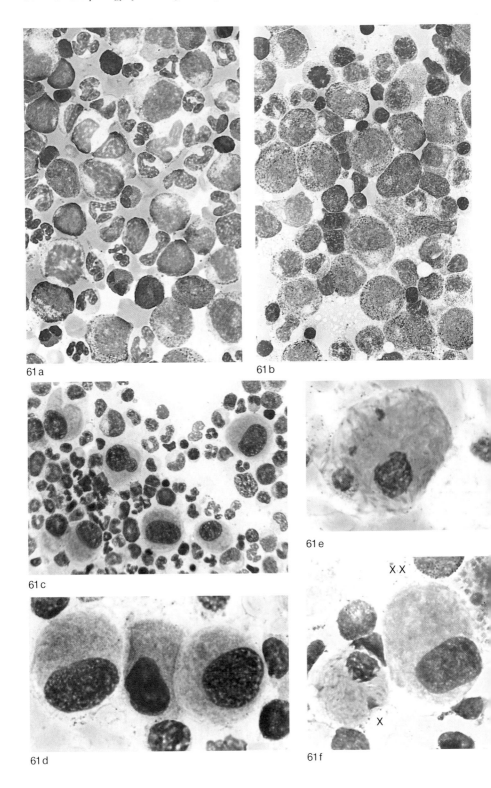

61 a

61 b

61 c

61 e

61 d

61 f

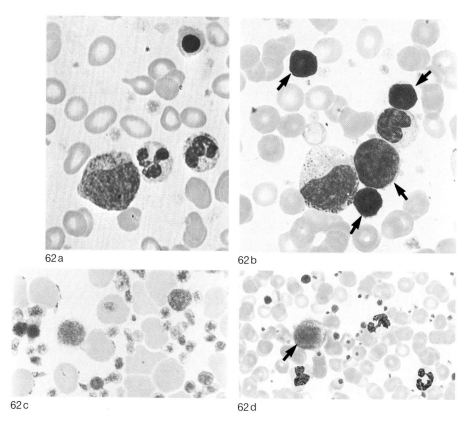

62 a

62 b

62 c

62 d

Fig. 62. Myeloproliferative diseases (blood smear/buffy coat). **a,** Myelofibrosis: anisopoikilocytosis of erythrocytes, leukemoid reaction (alongside two granulocytes and one promyelocyte; top, a normoblast); **b,** Same as **a,** nuclear fragments from megakaryocytes (arrows); **c–d,** Megakaryocytic myelosis (essential thrombocythemia): thrombocytosis with macrothrombocytes. **d,** Giant macrothrombocyte (arrow), large cell surrounded by granulocytes.

Fig. 61. Chronic myelocytic leukemia (bone marrow). **a,** Typical cell picture of stage II, increase in eosinophils and basophils, higher ME ratio (overview). **b,** For comparison with **a,** reactive granulopoiesis with inflammatory processes. **c,** Typical suppression of thrombopoiesis (microkaryocytes present) (overview). **d,** Microkaryocytes (markedly enlarged). **e,** A pseudo-Gaucher cell in the bone marrow in CML, stage II (rarely seen); no relation to Gaucher's disease (see Fig. 67h). **f,** Pseudo-Gaucher cell **(x)** next to a large microkaryocyte **(xx).**

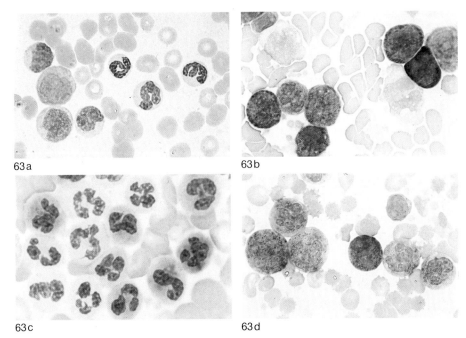

63a   63b

63c   63d

Fig. 63. Differential-diagnostic significance and diagnostic evaluation of leukocyte alkaline phosphatase (ALP).   **a,** Blood smear in chronic myelocytic leukemia; the enzyme activity is low in all mature granulocytes (stage I and II, mostly also in stage II–III). In stage III, the ALP activity can increase again in a few of the granulocytes present.   **b,** Higher activity index of ALP; often seen in polycythemia vera (in contrast to symptomatic macroglobulinemia) and in other diseases (see p. 111).   **c,** Normal ALP activity index (grade 0 to 2).   **d,** Middle grade (2 to 4) ALP activity index; significant increase seen in inflammatory granulocytosis (in contrast to **a**).   Note: For the classification and technique of leukocyte alkaline phosphatase, see p. 44 and p. 112, respectively. ALP indices (or scores) are determined only on blood smears.

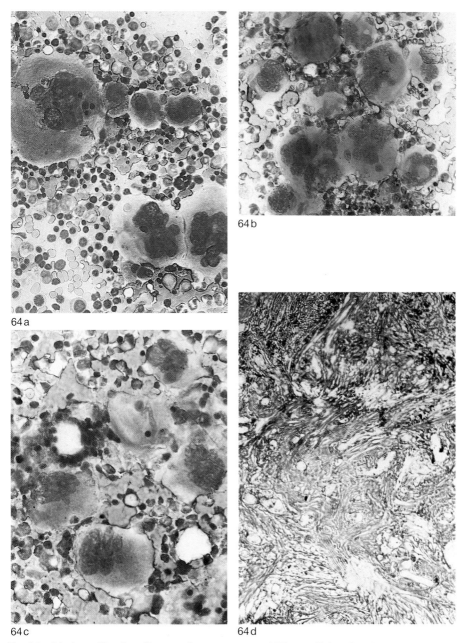

64b

64a

64c   64d

Fig. 64. Myeloproliferative diseases (bone marrow ×120). **a,** Polycythemia vera: increased granulopoiesis and thrombopoiesis along with increased erythropoiesis (panmyelosis), with bizarre nuclei in some megakaryocytes. No fat cells or iron storage.   **b,** Megakaryocytic myelosis: many bizarre-shaped megakaryocytes. **c,** Myelofibrotic syndrome: early stage, similar to **b. d,** End stage of disease: total fibrosis of the bone marrow; blood cell formation completely eliminated (Gomori stain; courtesy of Prof. Lennert, Kiel).

5.4   Morphologic Changes in Thrombopoiesis in Disease

Thrombocytoses may be a part of myeloproliferative diseases (pp. 71–77) or may be observed after splenectomy. Isolated thrombocytopenia must be considered as a specific disease entity as long as it is not associated with other hematopoietic disorders.

The principal causes of thrombocytopenia are as follows:

1. Infection, in particular viral infections in children (transitory thrombocytopenia).
2. Autoimmune platelet antibodies (principal cause of immune thrombocytopenia purpura [ITP]).
3. Drug-induced platelet antibodies. Thrombocytopenia of hypersplenism, systemic lupus erythematosus, Evans' syndrome (ITP with autoimmune hemolytic anemia), and acute leukemia are usually associated with advanced cytopenia or with changes of blood or bone marrow.

The morphologic diagnosis is principally for postinfection thrombocytopenia and ITP that exhibit characteristic compensating megakaryocytosis with or without significant left shift.

Note: See sections on pernicious anemia, myelodysplasia (pp. 57–59), chronic myeloid leukemia (pp. 72–75), and myelofibrosis (p. 75) for other pathologic changes in megakaryocytes. A thrombopenia can be induced with heparin.

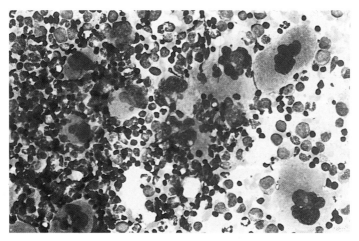

Fig. 65.   Typical picture of bone marrow in immune thrombocytopenia purpura (ITP) (essential thrombocytopenia), with clear compensating mega- (promega-) karyocytosis ($\times$120).

Fig. 66.   Bone marrow in isolated thrombocytopenia.   **a–d,** ITP: example of megakaryocytes that, in principle, cannot be distinguished from active thrombopoietic cells in normal bone marrow; **a** shows two promegakaryocytes, **d** shows weak PAS-positive reaction.   **e–f,** Clear vacuolization of megakaryocytes (through viral infection).

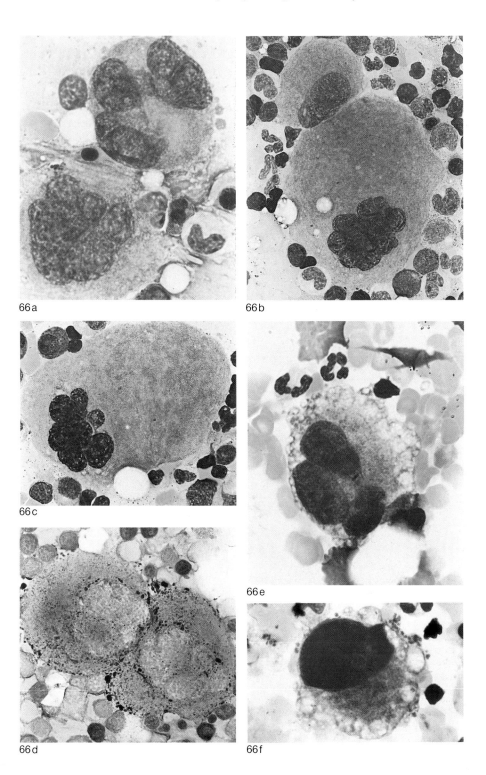

66a

66b

66c

66d

66e

66f

5.5   Morphologic Changes in the Reticuloendothelial System (RES, MMS) in Disease

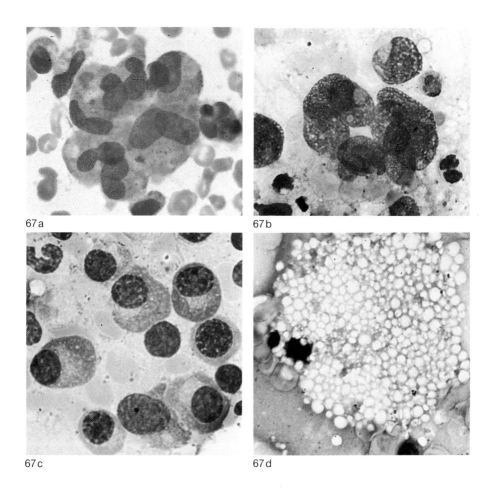

67a

67b

67c

67d

Fig. 67. Morphologic changes in the reticuloendothelial system. **a,** Endothelial phagocytosis in septic processes, particularly in bacterial endocarditis (rarely seen). **b,** Formation of granuloma in bone marrow or lymph nodes, e.g., in Boeck's sarcoidosis. The granuloma cells are formed from histiomonocytes. **c,** Plasma cellular reaction in bone marrow (plasmacytosis). Characteristic finding in diseases characterized by dysproteinemia, e.g., cirrhosis of the liver, nephrosis, and amyloidosis. **d,** Cholesterol storage in the bone marrow (Zieve syndrome). **e,** Precursor of storage cells in the bone marrow in early remission of AMoL ($\times$400). **f,** Higher magnification of storage cells in **e** ($\times$1200), probably swollen fat-storage histiomonocyte. **g,** Bone marrow in Niemann-Pick disease; swelling and drop formation in reticulum cells following sphingomyelin storage. **h,** Bone marrow in Gaucher's disease; major findings similar to those in **g,** but the storage products are glucocerebrosides (kerasin) and have a needle-shaped form.

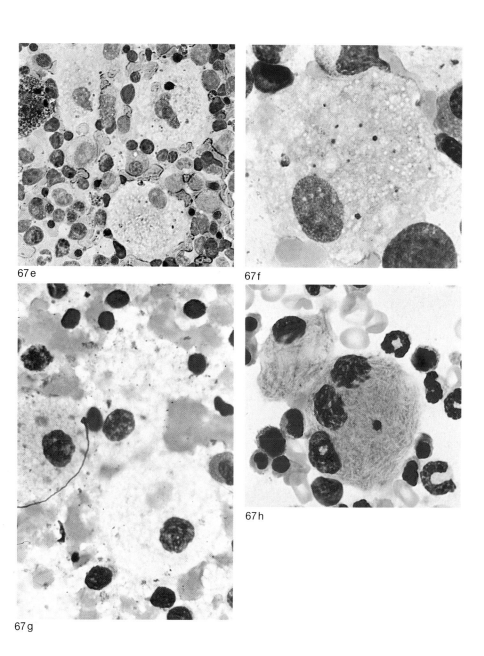

67 e

67 f

67 g

67 h

5.5.1   Rare Diseases in Bone Marrow Aspirates

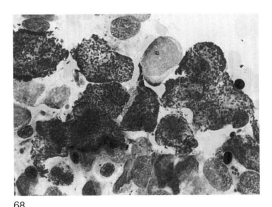

68

Fig. 68. Mast cell reticulocytosis. Malignancy of tissue mast cells, often accompanied by humoral symptoms (×1000).

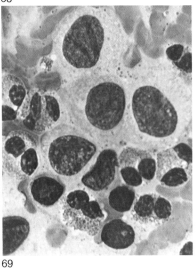

69

Fig. 69. Eosinophilic granuloma. Typical view, histiocytic elements alongside eosinophilic granulocytes. The same (monocytic) histiocytes are present in the rarely seen malignant histiocytosis.

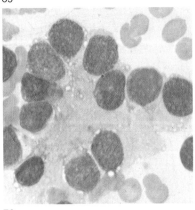

70

Fig. 70. Ewing's sarcoma. Typical tumor cell aggregation, with striking (very specific) vacuolization of the cytoplasm.

5.6   Morphologic Changes in Lymphopoiesis in Disease

5.6.1   Reactive Lymphocytosis

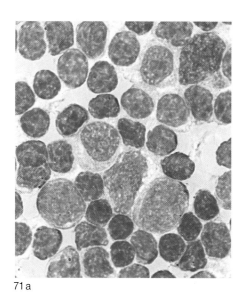

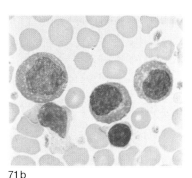

71 b

71 a

Fig. 71. a, Mixed lymphocytic response in lymph nodes (touch preparation) in nonspecific lymphadenopathy, also in toxoplasmosis.   **b,** Plasmablastic plasma cell reaction in rubeola (buffy coat).

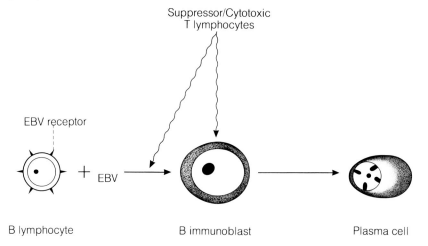

Fig. 72.   Immunologic processes in lymph nodes in infectious mononucleosis. B-lymphocytes are stimulated to produce B cell immunoblasts as a result of infection by the Epstein-Barr virus (EBV). The immunoblasts mature to plasma cells. Suppressor and cytotoxic T-lymphocytes stop this process and interrupt the virus infection of the B-lymphocytes (see Fig. 25c).

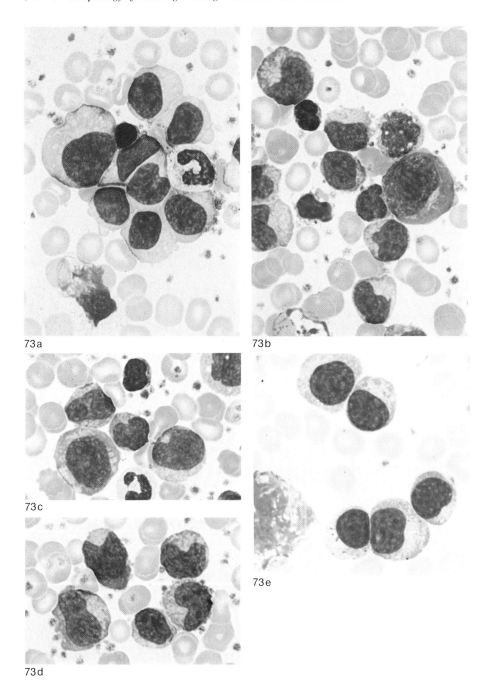

73a

73b

73c

73e

73d

Fig. 73. Infectious mononucleosis (peripheral blood or buffy coat smear). **a–c,** Typical lymphoid cell picture, with single large immunoblasts. **d,** Monocytic-type lymphoid cells (frequent observation). **e,** Lymphoid cells with partial beginning of autogranulation (suppressor cells). Note: The nuclear shape in lymphoid cells changes rapidly in EDTA blood.

5.6.2 Non-Hodgkin's Lymphoma (NHL, Kiel Classification)

Table 10. Kiel Classification of Non-Hodgkin's Lymphoma (1988)

B Cell Lymphoma	T Cells Lymphoma
Low-level malignant lymphomas	
Lymphocytic	Lymphocytic
Chronic lymphocytic leukemia*	Chronic lymphocytic leukemia†
Prolymphocytic leukemia*	Prolymphocytic leukemia†
Hairy cell leukemia*	Small cell ceribriform
	Mycosis fungoides, Sézary syndrome*
Lymphoplasmacytic/lymphoplasmacytoid (immunocytoma)*	Lymphoepithelioid (Lennert's lymphoma)
Plasmacytic*	Angioimmunoblastic (AILD, LgrX)
Centroblastic–centrocytic*	T-zone lymphoma
Follicular ± diffuse	
Diffuse	
Centrocytic	Pleomorphic, small cell (HTLV-I ±)
High malignancy lymphomas	
Centroblastic*	Pleomorphic, midsize to large cells (HTLV-I ±)
Immunoblastic*	Immunoblastic (HTLV-I ±)
Large cell, anaplastic (Ki-1 +)	Large cell, anaplastic (Ki-1 +)
Burkitt's lymphoma	
Lymphoblastic	Lymphoblastic*
Rare type	*Rare type*

* Cytologic diagnosis may be made from a lymph node preparation.
† Cytochemical diagnosis may be made from a lymph node preparation. (All other forms can be identified only by using immunohistologic procedures.)

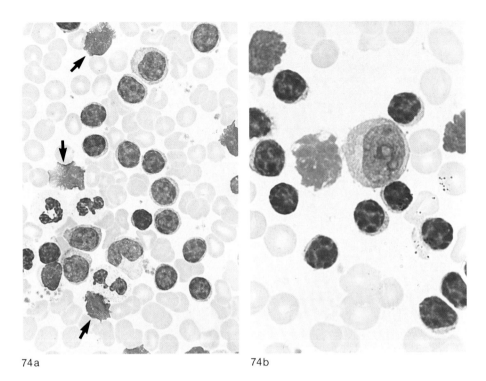

74a   74b

Fig. 74. Chronic lymphocytic leukemia (CLL). **a,** Typical picture in peripheral blood (overview): evident increase in the number of small lymphocytes (up to 500 × 10⁹/L are possible). Acute and subleukemic forms occur. Arrows show crushed lymphoblasts (damaged during the smearing technique), a typical sign of the fragility of lymphocytic leukemia cells (1) Prolymphocyte; (2) fragile immunoblast; (3) monocyte. **b,** Peripheral blood smear: a blastoid cell (lymphocyte) alongside mature lymphocytes.

Fig. 75. B-Cell chronic lymphocytic leukemia (CLL). **a,** Blastoid cells, as in Fig. 74b. **b,** Particularly large blast form in the peripheral blood in CLL (paraimmunoblast). **c,** Bone marrow aspirate in CLL (overview): along with the increase in the number of lymphocytes, many of the elements of myelopoiesis are evident (a sign of the relatively mild form of the disease). **d,** Bone marrow aspirate (touch preparation) in CLL: distinct lymphatic cell infiltration, comprised of small lymphocytes, one prolymphocyte (arrow), and one normoblast **(X).** A diffuse lymphocytic infiltration of the marrow is frequently evident, even when there are not yet any indications of a so-called suppression myelopathy (see Table 11). (**a** and **b,** ×1400). Note: Marrow lymphocytoses also occur in the absence of lymphocytic leukemia and immunocytoses, e.g., in myelopathies, autoimmune diseases, and juvenile iron deficiency. Also, part of an accidently aspirated normal or reactive (enlarged) marrow lymph node will give the impression of a diffuse lymphatic marrow infiltrate (see Fig. 29d).

Table 11.   RAI Classification of Chronic Lymphatic Leukemia (1975)

Stage 0	Blood lymphocyte count >15 × 10⁹/L
	Bone marrow lymphocytes: >40%
Stage I	Stage 0 + lymph node enlargement
Stage II	Stage 0 + splenomegaly and/or hepatomegaly (with or without lymph node enlargement)
Stage III	Stage 0 + anemia (blood hemoglobin concentration <110 g/L; with or without spleen, liver or lymph node enlargement)
Stage IV	Stage 0 + thrombopenia (platelets <100 × 10⁹/L) independent of hemoglobin level and/or spleen, liver, or lymph node enlargement.

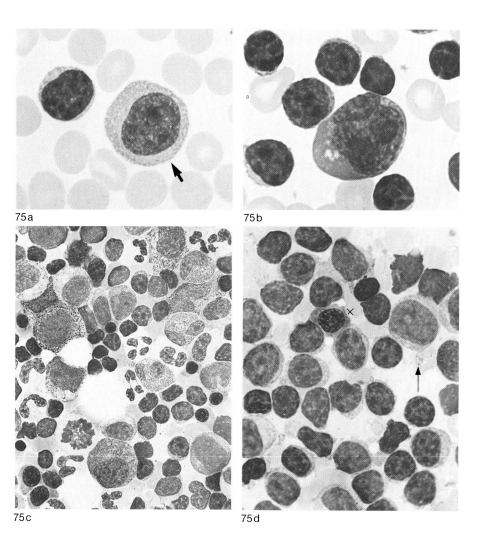

75a

75b

75c

75d

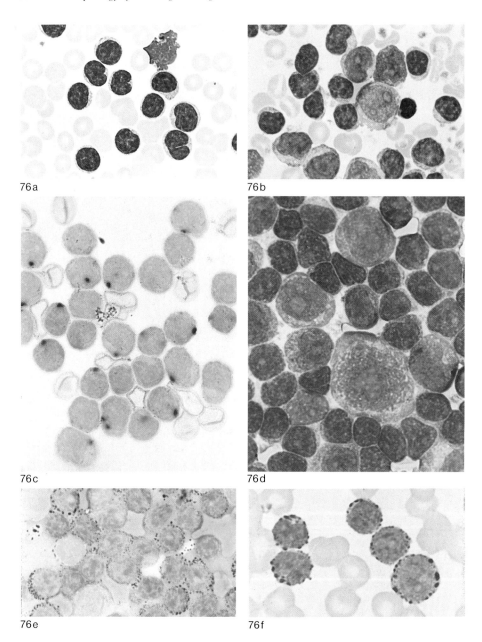

Fig. 76. Chronic lymphocytic leukemia (CLL).   **a,** Peripheral blood smear: partly crenated lymphocytes, in B-CLL (formerly called B₂-CLL).   **b,** Peripheral blood smear: advanced stage of CLL, with markedly atypical lymphocytic cell elements (**a** and **b,** ×500).   **c,** Peripheral blood smear: T-CLL, recognizable here by focal acid esterase activity.   **d,** Lymph node preparation: strikingly marked proliferative CLL. Alongside small lymphocytes are an increased number of immunoblasts (confirmed histologically).   **e,** Marrow smear: compared with the normal, the glycogen content of lymphocytes is increased in CLL (PAS stain).   **f,** Peripheral blood smear: particularly strong PAS staining in the final stage of CLL.   Note: The transition of a CLL to a centroblastic or immunoblastic lymphoma is the rarely seen Richter syndrome.

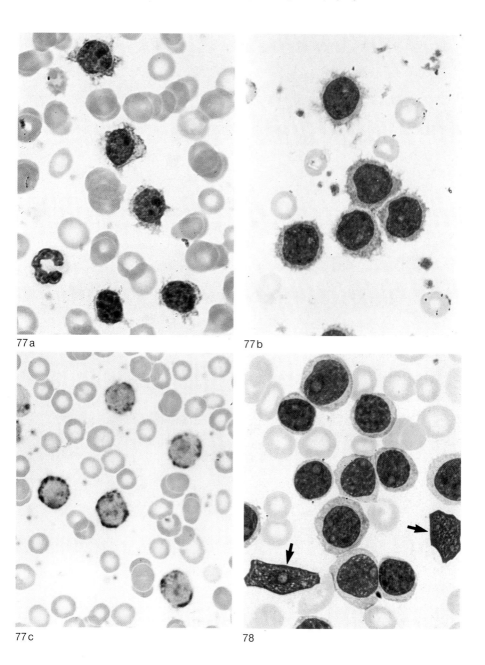

77a

77b

77c

78

Fig. 77. "Hairy cell leukemia" (HCL). **a–b,** Typical cell findings in the peripheral blood smear. **c,** Tartrate-resistant acid phosphatase in hairy cells (not a required criterion for making such a diagnosis).

Fig. 78. Prolymphocytic leukemia. Almost uniform, blast-like atypia of the markedly increased lymphocytic elements in a peripheral blood smear. Sometimes the same cytochemical observations as in hairy cells are seen. Arrows show damaged cells.

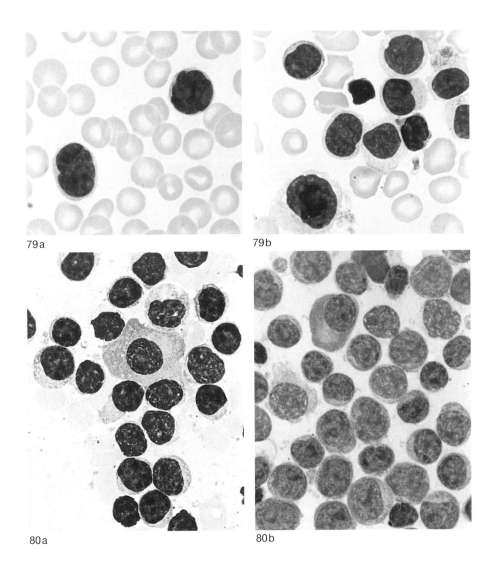

79a   79b

80a   80b

Fig. 79.   Sézary syndrome with mycosis fungoides. Typical cerebriform cells in the peripheral blood smear (morphologically altered T helper cells). A rare observation (Figure 79a courtesy of Prof. Löffler, Kiel.)

Fig. 80.   Lymphoplasmacytoid/plasmacytic immunocytoma (LPI).   **a,** Type of Waldenström's macroglobulinemia: preponderance of small lymphocytes and only a small increase in the number of plasma cells in the bone marrow next to sometimes increased marrow mast cells.   **b,** LPI: typical findings in a lymph node preparation.   **c,** Lymphoplasmacytoid immunocytoma: in-

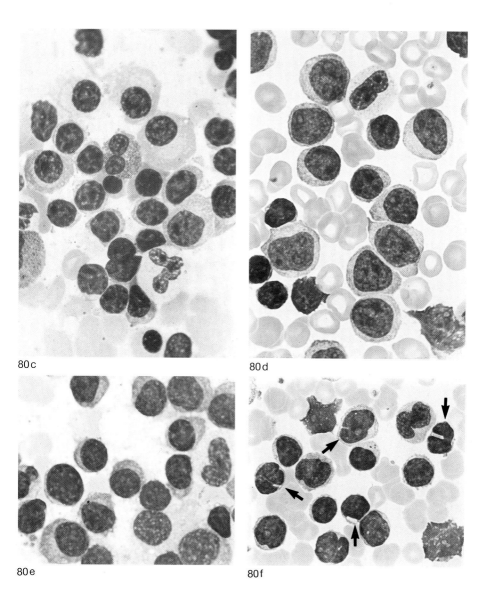

80c

80d

80e

80f

crease in lymphocytes mixed with plasma cells (bone marrow). **d,** Polymorphic immunocytoma (monoclonal IgM-gammopathy) (buffy coat preparation): leukemic flow of blastoid and plasmacytic elements into the peripheral blood. **e,** Immunocytoma with clear plasmacytic components (bone marrow). **f,** LPI (leukocyte concentrate): crystalline protein inclusions in lymphocytes. Note: A definite differential diagnosis between LPI and CLL can be made only immunohistochemically.

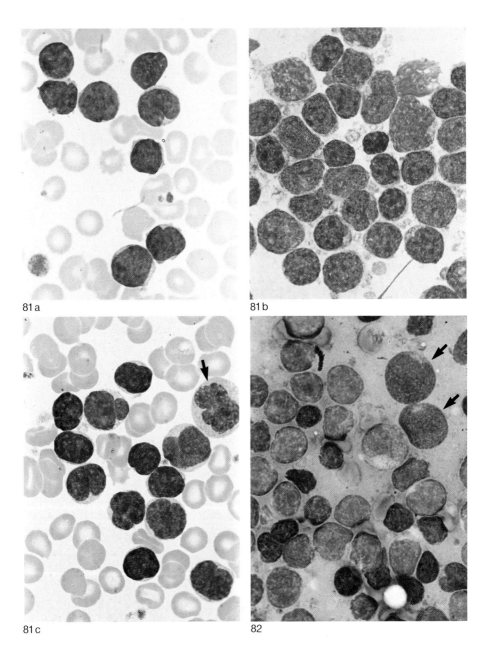

81 a   81 b

81 c   82

Fig. 81.   Centrocytic non-Hodgkin's lymphoma (NHL).   **a,** Typical crenated cells (cleaved cells) in a buffy coat preparation.   **b,** Centrocytic NHL in a lymph node preparation with clear beginning of undifferentiation.   **c,** Buffy coat preparation: anaplastic centrocytic NHL (cell elements with considerable morphologically recognizable malignancy). Arrow shows monocyte. (Histology corroborated by Prof. Lennert, Kiel.)

Fig. 82.   Centroblastic-centrocytic NHL.   Typical cytology of a lymph node biopsy. Arrows show centroblasts. In contrast to Figure 81, a less active cell picture. (Histology by Prof. Lennert, Kiel.)

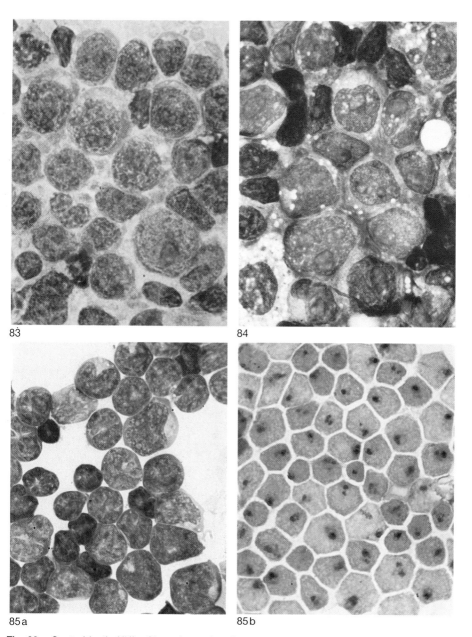

83
84
85a
85b

Fig. 83. Centroblastic NHL. Clear signs of malignancy, lymph node biopsy preparation. (Histology corroborated by Prof. Lennert, Kiel.)

Fig. 84. Immunoblastic NHL. Lymph node biopsy preparation. (Histology corroborated by Prof. Lennert, Kiel.)

Fig. 85. T-lymphoblastic NHL, early convoluted type. **a,** Centrifuged sediment of pleural exudate; Wright's stain. **b,** Same as **a,** with typical focal reaction with acid phosphatase stain. Note: For lymphoblastic leukemia, see pp. 68–69.

5.6.3   Hodgkin's Lymphoma

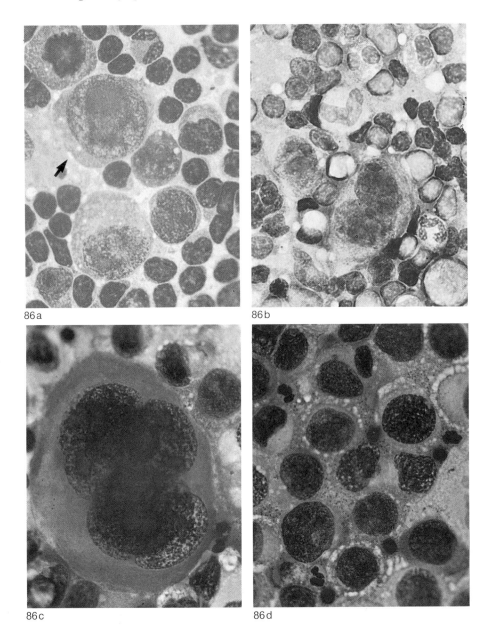

86a

86b

86c

86d

Fig. 86.   Hodgkin's lymphoma.   **a,** Early changes in a lymph node biopsy preparation. Arrow shows young Hodgkin's cell.   **b,** Typical picture of lymph node cells, showing Reed-Sternberg cells and eosinophils ($\times$400).   **c,** Reed-Sternberg–like giant cells.   **d,** So-called Hodgkin's sarcoma, with clear morphologic similarities to giant cell anaplastic (Ki-1 +) lymphoma (see Table 10, p. 85).   Note: Observation of specific Hodgkin's elements in a bone marrow aspirate is rare.

5.6.4 Plasmacytoma

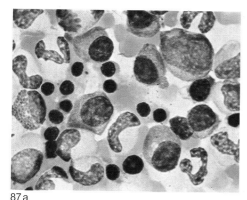

87a

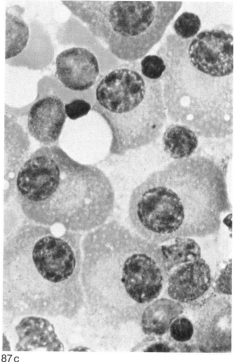

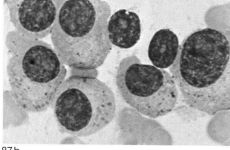

87b

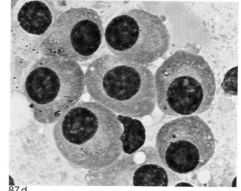

87c

Fig. 87. Plasmacytoma (multiple myeloma, Kahler's disease). **a,** Early plasmacytoma, positive indications on immunoelectrophoresis: discrete small changes in the nucleus of the significantly increased number of plasma cells (confirmed by monitoring changes). **b,** Bone marrow aspirate: many undifferentiated plasma cells (plasmacytoma cells) in Bence-Jones plasmacytoma. The cytoplasm has azurophilic granulation (rare). **c,** Bone marrow aspirate: broad cytoplasmic elements with large immature cell nucleus (loss of the typical coarse chromatin structure of normal plasma cells); nucleoli evident. Seen in IgA plasmacytoma. **d,** Bone marrow aspirate: IgG plasmacytoma. Degree of undifferentiation less than that in **b** and **c.** **e,** Plasmacytoma cells with characteristic Russell body formation.

87d

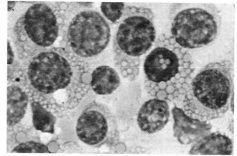

87e

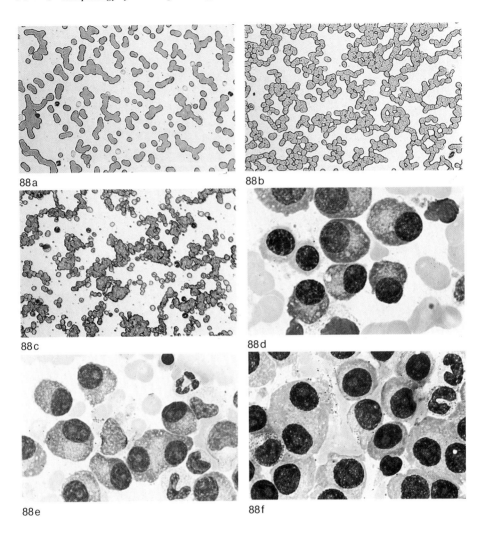

88a

88b

88c

88d

88e

88f

Fig. 88. Plasmacytoma. **a,** Typical rouleaux formation of erythrocyte aggregation (pseudoagglutination) in a monoclonal gammopathy. **b,** Erythrocyte aggregation as a result of an increase in α_2-globulin and fibrinogen. **c,** Erythrocyte agglutination with autoimmunohemolysis. (Compare **b** and **c** with **a**.) **d,** Plasmacytoma cells in a relatively mild case of the disease. **e,** Plasmacytoma cells in intermediate degree of malignant disease (nucleoli positive). **f,** Plasmacytoma cells in highly malignant disease. **g,** Multinucleated plasmacytoma cell. **h,** Strongly positive acid phosphatase reaction in plasmacytoma cells (typical but not specific). **i,** "Flaming" plasmacytoma cell (mostly IgA type). **k,** Peripheral blood smear:

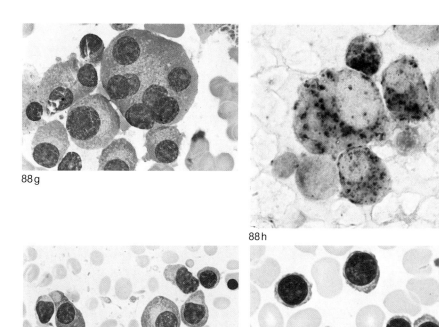

88g

88h

88i

88k

plasma cell leukemia (the typical displacement of the plasma cell nucleus is lost in favor of the lymphatic cell characteristics).   Note: There is no good correlation between immunoelectrophoretic findings and the morphology of the plasmacytoma cells. One can establish, independently of the morphologic picture, a decreasing scale of malignancy: IgD, Bence-Jones, IgA, IgG. The morphologic picture, however, gives a good indication of the long-term prognosis for the disease. IgM-plasmacytomas are lymphoplasmacytic immunocytomas—cases of Waldenström's macroglobulinemia or rarer diseases. Benign monoclonal gammopathies have no specific pathologic cell characteristics; they can transform into plasmacytomas.

6 Appendix

6.1 Cancer Cells in Bone Marrow Aspirates

The detection of cancer cells in the bone marrow aspirate of metastatic neoplasms occurs less frequently than might be expected from the actual participation of the bone marrow in the metastatic process. A bone marrow biopsy, however, should be carried out in all cases of suspected tumors and in neoplasms that appear to be responsive to treatment. A primary condition for the highest possible yield is an optimal tapping and smear technique. The nest-shaped arrangement of tumor cells in the marrow smears must be considered as a typical useful diagnostic positive microscopic result (see Fig. 89a). Only in rare cases can conclusions be drawn about the primary site of the tumor from the cytomorphologic properties of the individual carcinoma cells, particularly because every neoplastic cell picture is different.

In Figure 89, the individual organ diagnoses were histologically confirmed. For indication of the leukemoid blood reaction in bone marrow carcinoma, see p. 64.

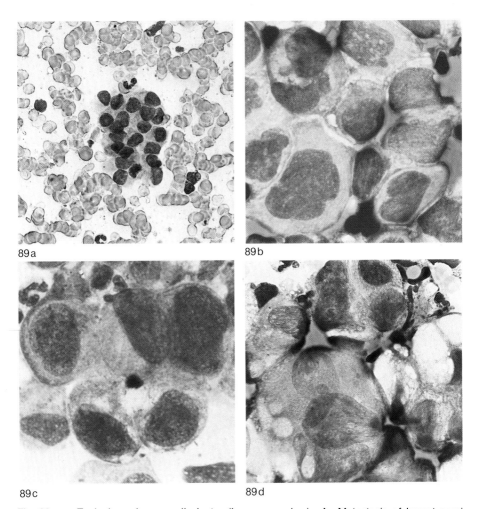

89a

89b

89c

89d

Fig. 89.   a, Typical carcinoma cell cluster (low-power view).   **b,** Metastasis of breast carcinoma.   **c,** Large cell bronchogenic carcinoma.   **d,** Mucinous/colloidal carcinoma of the intestinal tract.   **e,** Metastasis of a melanoma.   **f,** Metastasis of an ovarian carcinoma (cells are somewhat necrotic).   **g,** Metastasis of a renal cell carcinoma (hypernephroma) (low-power view). (**g** and **h,** × 1200.)

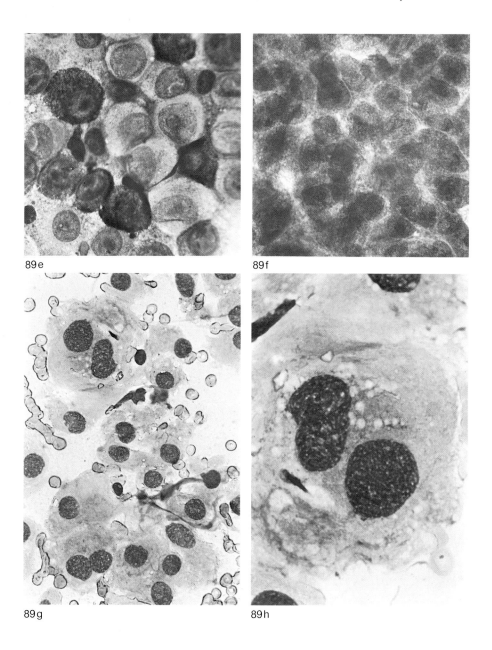

89 e

89 f

89 g

89 h

6.2   Phases of Mitosis in Bone Marrow Aspirates

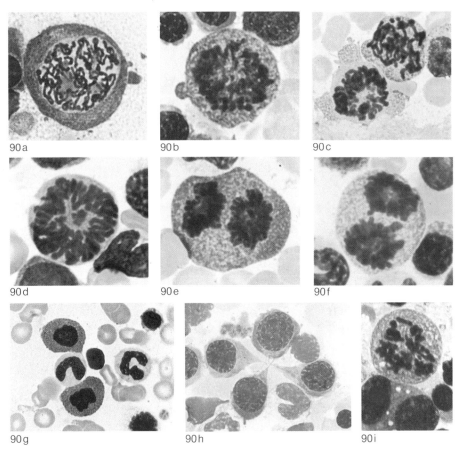

90 a   90 b   90 c

90 d   90 e   90 f

90 g   90 h   90 i

Fig. 90.   Phases of mitosis in the bone marrow.   **a,** Stage I: prophase (megaloblast).   **b,** Stage II: late metaphase (proerythroblast).   **c,** Late and early metaphase in two carcinoma cells.   **d,** Stage II: late metaphase (myeloblast).   **e,** Stage III: anaphase (proerythroblast with numerous mitochondria).   **f,** Stage III: anaphase (promyelocyte or promonocyte).   **g,** Stage IV: telophase (eosinophilic myelocyte); two daughter cells without full rebuilding of the nucleus; between them, a band nucleus.   **h,** Completed telophase (2 × 2 daughter cells, basophilic normoblasts). Complete rebuilding of the nucleus. Fine thread-like cytoplasmic bridges cross between pairs of cells (incidental finding).   **i,** Multipolar endomitosis in a Hodgkin's cell, preliminary to the development of Reed-Sternberg cells (lymph node biopsy).

6.3   Instructions for the Evaluation of Bone Marrow Aspirates

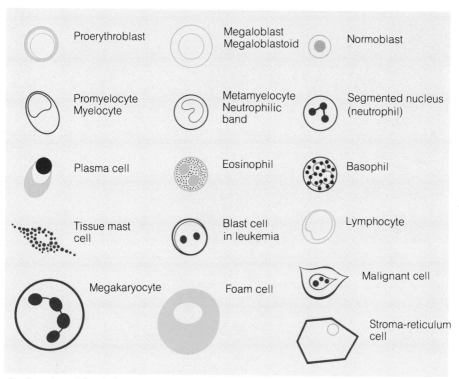

Explanation of Symbols

6.3.1   Determination of Cellularity

Technical Prerequisite.   Well-spread marrow material, magnifications × 100 and × 400.

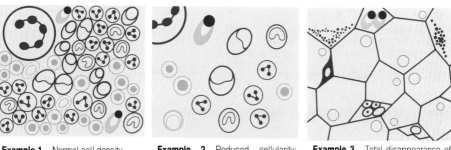

Example 1.   Normal cell density.

Example 2.   Reduced cellularity; large source of error in assessment of the true marrow situation (can be caused technically by having a poor aspirate containing a mixture of blood).

Example 3.   Total disappearance of hematopoietic cells (empty marrow, consisting of stroma, fat, plasma, and tissue mast cells and reticulum elements).

6.3.2   Determination of Qualitative Composition

Technical Prerequisite.   Well-spread marrow material, magnifications × 100, × 400, and oil immersion.

Erythropoiesis (EP)

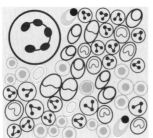

Example 1. Normal EP, normal maturation of all systems. Proportion of granulopoiesis to EP (ME ratio) = 3.5.

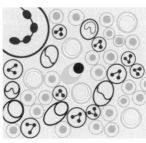

Example 2. Increased maturing EP (e.g., in hemorrhagic anemia).

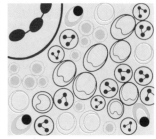

Example 3. Partially increased EP, partially inconspicuous (e.g., in iron deficiency anemia without a regenerating component or in anemia resulting from infection).   (Differential   diagnosis: stored iron.)

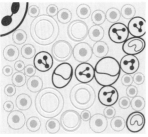

Example 4. Grossly increased EP with good maturation. Typical for hemolytic anemia. ME ratio <1.

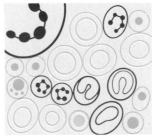

Example 5. Grossly increased EP with well-marked megaloblastosis, giant nuclei (either erythroid or myeloid), and hypersegmentation of neutrophils. Typical for pernicious anemia.

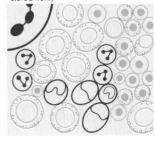

Example 6. Grossly increased megaloblastic EP, with left shift. In this example, sideroachrestic anemia (with iron-stain–positive ring sideroblasts).

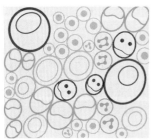

Example 7. Increased, mostly megaloblastic, EP; increase in number of microkaryocytes. Typical for myelodysplasia.

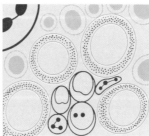

Example 8. Malignant degeneration of EP, with PAS-positive erythroblasts (Di Guglielmo disease).

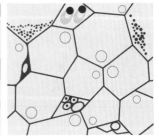

Example 9. Absence of EP. Aplastic anemia as a partial symptom of pancytopenias.

Granulopoiesis (GrP)

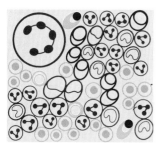

Example 1. Normal GrP (ME ratio = 3.5).

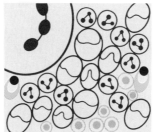

Example 2. Increased GrP, maturing. Typical for infections, necrosis, and Hodgkin's disease. ME ratio >5.5. Peripheral blood: granulocytosis with moderate left shift.

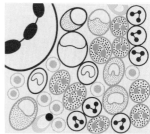

Example 3. Increased GrP; maturing, strongly eosinophilic. Typical for allergic reaction.

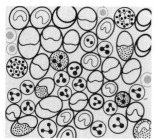

Example 4. Grossly increased GrP with left shift (typical for chronic myelocytic leukemia), accompanied by increased numbers of eosinophils and basophils. Peripheral blood: marked granulocytosis with left shift up to promyelocytes.

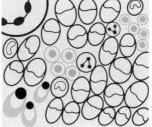

Example 5. Increased GrP with left shift; promyelocytic marrow. Typical for agranulocytosis. Peripheral blood: usually leukopenia.

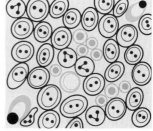

Example 6. Displaced GrP with infiltration of the blast. Typical for acute leukemia.

Thrombopoiesis (ThrP)

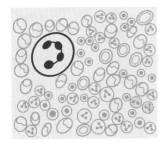 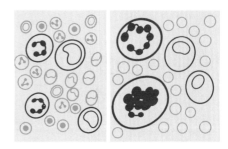

Example 1. Normal ThrP (× 100); 1 megakaryocyte in every 4th to 6th field of view (1 to 5 per 1000 marrow cells).

Example 2. Left, Increased ThrP, eventually with increasing numbers of often atypical promegakaryocytes. Characteristic of idiopathic (autoimmune) thrombocytopenia purpura.   Right, Increase in atypical megakaryocytes in myeloproliferative diseases (microkaryocytes in myelodysplasia and CML, bizarre nuclei in megakaryocytic myelosis and myelofibrosis).

Reticuloendothelial System (RES, MMS) and Lymphopoiesis

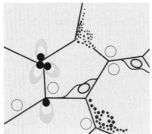 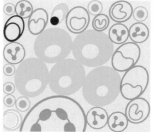 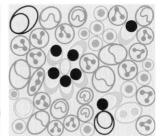

Example 1. Reactive multiplication of the reticulum elements with disappearance of the blood-forming tissues. Typical of panmyelophthisis.

Example 2. Increase in number of lipid-storing reticulum cells. Typical for Niemann-Pick, Gaucher's, and Hand-Schüller-Christian diseases, Zieve syndrome, and toxic marrow damage.

Example 3. Plasmacytic reaction. Typical of dysproteinemic or inflammatory disease.

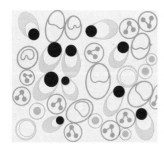 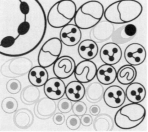 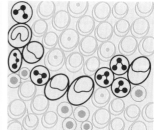

Example 4. Tumor-like proliferation of the plasma cells. Typical of plasmacytoma.

Example 5. Normal marrow, with only small interspersion of lymphocytes (from peripheral blood or lymph follicles of the marrow); discrete, mostly focal marrow lymphocytosis. Found particularly in immunologic diseases or in marrow aplasia.

Example 6. Lymphocytic infiltration, consisting predominantly of small lymphocytes, which successively displace normal hemopoiesis; typical of marrow participation in CLL.

Neoplasias

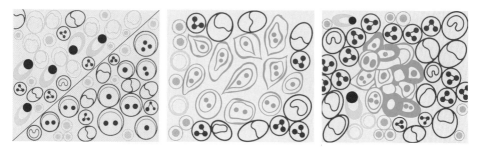

Example 1. Marrow in non-Hodgkin's lymphoma. **a,** Immunocytoma. **b,** Lymphoblastic lymphoma.

Example 2. Proliferation of tumor cells in Ewing's sarcoma, hairy cell leukemia, or malignant histiocytosis.

Example 3. Metastatic carcinoma in the bone marrow (for comparison).

Note: Bone marrow aspirates of the sternum or the pelvis cannot, in all pathologic cases, be considered as representative of the condition of the bone marrow; focal changes sometimes can escape detection by the morphologic method. Additional examination of the marrow of the pelvis or a Jamshidi aspirate is recommended.

A Technique for Bone Marrow Imprints from a Bone Marrow Aspirate or a Postmortem Special Specimen

Procedure

1. On the center of a clean glass slide, add a drop of bone marrow aspirate, or place the marrow particle (postmortem specimen) on a piece of cardboard and then lightly touch the top of the particle with a glass slide.
2. Place the glass slide on the table, and place another clean glass slide on the top of the first slide.
3. Let the marrow spread; then apply light pressure to the top of the covering glass slide. The marrow will spread further.
4. Separate the slides by lifting the top slide. (Freeing the slides by sliding apart should be avoided.)
5. Air-dry, fix, and stain as for any peripheral blood smear, or as described for the special stains (pp. 112–118).

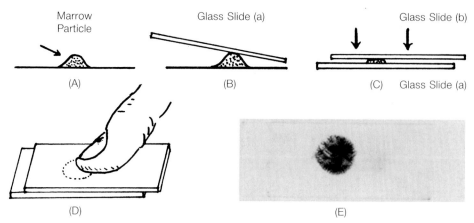

Fig. 91. Technique for making the imprint: The bone marrow particle is placed on a piece of cardboard **(A).** Lightly touch the top of the particle with a glass slide **(B),** and place a second slide on the first glass slide **(C).** Add light pressure evenly on the glass slide **(b),** using an index finger **(D).** An actual marrow imprint after staining with Wright's stain **(E).** (Reproduced, by permission, from Kao: A Technic for Bone Marrow Imprints from Postmortem Specimen [1975]. Am J. Clin. Pathol. 63:833.)

6.3.3   Cytology and Histology

A comparison of findings from cytologic and histologic examinations in certain diseases is shown in Table 12, which should serve as a guide for their use. In all doubtful cases, a combination of cytologic and histologic examinations should be used, and for dry marrow aspirates, the fundamental histologic diagnosis should be given preference.

Table 12.   Comparison of Findings from Cytologic and Histologic Examinations. (Histologic findings courtesy of Prof. Lennert, Kiel, and Prof. Burkhardt, Munich.)

Diagnosis	Cytology*	Histology*
Anemia (general)	+ + +	rare
Aplastic anemia	+	+ +
Panmyelopathy	+	+ +
Preleukemia	+ +	(+)/ + (E)
Acute leukemia	+ + +	rare (E)
Chronic myelocytic leukemia	+	+
Polycythemia vera	+	+ +
Megakaryocytic myelosis, myelofibrosis	+ / −	+ + +
Non-Hodgkin's lymphoma		
Chronic lymphocytic leukemia	+	+
Hairy cell leukemia	(+)	+ +
Other forms	+ / + +	+ +
Plasmacytoma	+ + +	+ (E)
Hodgkin's lymphoma	− /(+)	+
Carinoma (metastatic)	+	+ +
Cytochemical iron	+	+
Other reactions	+ + +	rare

* (E), possible source of error; + + +, strong positive reaction; + +, positive reaction; +, weak positive reaction; (+), questionable positive reaction; −, no reaction.

6.3.4 List of Monoclonal Antibodies in Use in Diagnostic Hematology

Table 13. Classification of Monoclonal Antibodies*

CD Number	Monoclonal Antibodies	Reactivity
CD 1a	NA1/34, T6, VIT6, Leu6	Thy, DC, B-Subset
CD 1b	WM-25, 4A76, NUT2	Thy, DC, B-Subset
CD 1c	L161, M241, 7C6, PHM3	Thy, DC, B-Subset
CD 2	9.6, T11, 35.1	T
CD 2R	T11.3, VIT13, D66	Active T
CD 3	T3, UCHT1, 38.1, Leu4	T
CD 4	T4, Leu3a, 91.D6	T-Subset
CD 5	T1, UCHT2, T101, HH9, AMG4	T, B-Subset
CD 6	T12, T411	T, B-Subset
CD 7	3A1, 4A, CL1.3, G3–7	T
CD 8	α-chain: T8, Leu2a, M236, UCHT4, T811	T-Subset
	β-chain: T8/2T8–5H7	
CD 9	CLB-thromb/8, PHN200, FMC56	Pre-B, M, Plt
CD 10	J5, VILA1, BA-3	Lymphat. precursor, cALL Germ center B, G
CD 11a	MHM24, 2F12, CRIS-3	Leukocyte
CD 11b	Mo1, 5A4.C5, LPM19C	M, G, NK
CD 11c	B-Ly6, L29, BL-4H4	M, G, NK, B-Subset
CD w12	M67	M, G, Plt
CD 13	MY7, MCS-2, TÜK 1, MOU28	M, G
CD 14	Mo2, UCHM1, VIM13, MoP15	M, (G), LHC
CD 15	My 1, VIM-D5	G, (M)
CD 16	BW209/2, HUNK2, VEP13, 3G8	NK, (G), macrophages
CD w17	GO35, Huly-m13	G, M, Plt
CD 18	MHM23, M232, 11H6, CLB54	Leukocytes
CD 19	B4, H37	B
CD 20	B1, 1F5	B
CD 21	B2, HB5	B-Subset
CD 22	HD39, S-HCL1, To15	Cytoplasmic B Surface-B-Subset
CD 23	Blast-2, MHM6	B-Subset, active M, Eo
CD 24	VIBE3, BA-1	B, G
CD 25	TAC, 7G7/B6, 2A3	Active T, B, M
CD 26	134-2C2, TS145	Active T
CD 27	VIT14, S152, OKT18A, CLB-9F4	T-Subset
CD 28	9.3, KOLT2	T-Subset
CD 29	K20, A-1A5	Wide
CD 30	Ki-1, Ber-H2, HSR4	Active T, B, Reed-Sternberg
CD 31	SG134, TM3, HEC-75, ES12F11	Plt, M, G, B, (T)
CD w32	CIKM5, 41H16, IV.3, 2E1, KB61	M, G, B, Plt
CD 33	My9, H153, L4F3	M, precursor AML
CD 34	My10, BI-3C5, ICH-3	Precursor cells
CD 35	TO5, CB04, J3D3	G, M, B
CD 36	5F1, CIMeg1, ESIVC7	M, Plt, (B)
CD 37	HD28, HH1, G28-1	B, (T, M)
CD 38	HB7, T16	Lymphat. precursor DC, active T
CD 39	AC2, G28-2	B-Subset, (M)
CD 40	G28-5	B, carcinoma cells
CD 41	PBM6.4, CLB-thromb/7, PL273	Plt

Table 13. (*continued*)

CD Number	Monoclonal Antibodies	Reactivity
CD 42a	FMC25, BL-H6, GR-P	Plt
CD 42b	PHN89, AN51, GN287	Plt
CD 43	OTH71C5, G19-1, MEM59	T, G, M, brain
CD 44	GRHL1, F10-44-2, 33-3B3, BRIC35	T, G, M, brain, Ery
CD 45	T29/33, BMAC1, AB187	Leukocytes
CD 45RA	G1-15, F8-11-13, 73.5	T-Subset, B, G, M
CD 45RB	PTD/26/16	T-Subset, B, G, M
CD 45RO	UCHL1	T-Subset, B, G, M
CD 46	HULYM5, 122-2, J4B	Leukocytes
CD 47	BRIC126, CIKM1, BRIC125	Wide
CD 48	WM68, LO-MN25, J4-57	Leukocytes
CD w49b	CLB-thromb/4, Gi14	Plt, cultured T cells
CD w49d	B5G10, HP2/1, HP1/3	M, T, B, (LHC), Thy
CD w49f	GoH3	Plt, (T)
CD w50	101-1D2, 140-11	Leukocytes
CD 51	13C2, 23C6, NKI-M7, NKI-M9	(Plt) (B)
CD w52	097, YTH66.9, Campath-1	Leukocytes
CD 53	MEM-53, HI29, HI36, HD77	Leukocytes
CD 54	RR7/7F7, WEHI-CAMI	Wide, activated cells
CD 55	143-30, BRIC 110, BRIC 128, F2B-7.2	Wide
CD 56	Leu19, NKH1, FP2-11.14, L185	NK, active lymphocytes
CD 57	Leu7, L183, L186	NK, T, B-Subset, brain
CD 58	TS2/9, G26, BRIC5	Leukocytes, epithelium
CD 59	YTH53.1, MEM-43	Wide
CD w60	M-T32, M-T21, M-T41, UM4D4	T-Subset
CD 61	Y2/51, CLB-thromb/1, VI-PL-2, BL-E6	Plt
CD 62	CLB-thromb/6, CLB-thromb/5, RUU-SP1.18.1	Active Plt
CD 63	RUU-SP2.28, CLB-gran/12	Active Plt, M, (G, T, B)
CD 64	Mab32.2, Mab22	M
CD w65	VIM2, HE10, CF4, VIM8	G, M
CD 66	CLBgran/10, YTH71.3	G
CD 67	B13.9, G10F5, JML-H16	G
CD 68	EBM11, Y2/131, Y-1/82A, Ki-M7, Ki-M6	Macrophages
CD 69	MLR-3, L78, BL-Ac/p26, FN50	Active B, T
CD w70	Ki-24, HNE 51, HNC 142	Active B, active T, Reed-Sternberg
CD 71	138-18, 120-2A3, MEM-75, VIP-1, Nu-Tfr2	Proliferating cells Macrophages
CD 72	S-HCL2, J3-109, BU-40, BU-41	B
CD 73	1E9.28.1, 7G2.2.11, AD2	B-Subset, T-Subset
CD 74	LN2, BU-43, BU-45	B, M
CD w75	LN1, HH2, EBU-141	Mature B, (T-Subset)
CD 76	HD66, CRIS-4	Mature B, T-Subset
CD 77	38.13(BLA), 424/4A11, 424/3D9	Differentiated B
CD w78	AntiBa, LO-panB-a, 1588	B, (M)

* With permission from Knapp, W. et al.: CD antigens 1989. Blood 74:1448 (1989).
Abbreviations: Thy = thymocyte; DC = dendritic reticulum cell; B = B-lymphocyte; T = T-lymphocyte; M = monocyte; G = granulocyte; Plt = thrombocyte; NK = natural killer cell.

6.4   Indications for Use of Cytochemical Procedures

Peroxidase (POX); Sudan Black B

a. Positive identification of the normal elements of granulopoiesis (except normal blast cells); monocytes give a positive reaction, but lymphatic cells are negative.

b. Classification of AML and AMML; particularly good reaction with Auer rods. Required procedure for the differential diagnosis of AML and ALL.

c. Exact evaluation of the elements of granulopoiesis in the remission of acute leukemias.

Nonspecific Esterase (Est.)

a. Positive identification of monocytes in contrast to their precursors. (Monocyte-forming macrophages also react positively.)

b. Classification of AMOL and AMML.

c. Acid esterase: classification of T-lymphocytes.

Leukocyte Alkaline Phosphatase (ALP)

Usefull for the following:

a. Reactive neutrophilia or granulocytoses.

b. Chronic myelocytic leukemias.

c. Myeloproliferative disorders.

d. Polycythemia vera (particularly the differential diagnosis with multiple myeloma).

e. Hairy cell leukemia (strong positive reaction of the granulocytes).

f. Monitoring of Hodgkin's and non-Hodgkin's lymphomas.

Periodic Acid-Schiff (PAS) Reaction

a. Good staining of mature granulocytes and basophils.

b. Indication of the different phases of the activity of megakaryocytes. Thrombocytes also react positively.

c. Glycogen synthesis in lymphocytes (used to monitor cell proliferation in CLL).

d. Positive reaction with cytoplasmic granules in certain forms of ALL (particularly c-ALL), in the lymphoid blast phase of CML. Positive reaction with individual or aggregated granules in the early stages of normoblasts in Di Guglielmo disease, occasionally in monoblasts in AMOL. Sometimes a diffuse reaction is seen in more mature normoblasts in Di Guglielmo disease and in Russell bodies in plasma cells.

Iron Reaction (Presence of Iron)

a. Determination of iron stores in bone marrow.

b. Evidence of physiologic and pathologic sideroblasts and siderocytes.

c. Detection of atypical or pathologic iron stores.

Acid Phosphatase (AP)

a. Distinguishing certain types of ALL from non-Hodgkin's lymphoma (T-ALL, T-lymphoblastic lymphoma).

b. Characterization of lymphocytes (granular or spotted reaction products).
c. Diagnostic aid for hairy cell leukemia and also for prolymphocytic leukemia (tartrate-resistant acid phosphatase reaction, not a conclusive observation).
d. Strong reaction in plasma cells, particularly strong in plasmocytoma cells.

Dipeptidylamino Peptidase (DAP IV)
Only for demonstration of the presence of T-lymphocytes (very specific, yet only positive in approximately 40% of T-ALL cases).

Toluidine Blue
For demonstration of specific granulation in blood and tissue basophils.

6.5   Preparation of Special Stains

6.5.1   Leukocyte Alkaline Phosphatase Reaction
(Kapłow/Merker method)

Staining Procedure
a. Fix air-dried blood smears (less than 3 days old) for 30 seconds at 4° C in a mixture of 90 parts absolute methanol (100%) and 10 parts formalin (37%).
b. Rinse in running water and air dry.
c. Incubate for 1 hour at 4 to 5° C (in a refrigerator) in freshly prepared staining solution made of 70 mg of variamine blue salt B conc. and 35 mg of sodium naphthyl-l-phosphate in 70 mL of sodium barbital (20 g/L) at pH 9.4. Filtration of the solution of diazonium salt in buffer is recommended before addition of the dissolved substrate.
d. Rinse in running water and air dry.
e. Stain the nucleus with Mayer's hematoxylin stain for 3 to 5 minutes.
f. Rinse and air dry.

Reaction Product.   Yellow-brown-black.

Counting.   The counting is done in the counting zone of the smear. One hundred (or a multiple) neutrophils, with band and segmented nuclei, are counted consecutively and classified from 0 to 4, according to the strength of their reaction with the stain. The total number of cells in each class, multiplied by its class factor, gives the activity number, or index, of the smear. (See also pp. 44, 76).

Reference range.   ALP index 10–100; maximum 400–500.

Reagents
Sodium barbital
Sodium naphthyl-l-phosphate
Variamine blue salt B (diazonium salt)

Preparation of the Substrate Mixture

a. Add 70 mg of variamine blue salt to 50 ml of 20 g/l barbital solution.
b. Add 35 mg of sodium naphthyl-l-phosphate to 20 ml of 20 g/l barbital solution.
c. Filter solutions (a) and (b) into the staining trough, cover, and store in a refrigerator.
   Note: Numerous formulations exist for the leukocyte alkaline phosphatase incubation mixture. Other diazo dyes can be used for this purpose. If blue diazo dye is used, red nuclear counterstaining is recommended.

6.5.2   Peroxidase Reaction
(POX reaction of Schäfer and Fischer without benzidine)

Staining Procedure

a. Use 24-hour specimens for preparation of smear.
b. Fix the air-dried smears for 30 seconds in filtered 10% (v/v) formaldehyde/alcohol solution and rinse immediately with tap water.
c. Staining solution: dissolve 10 mg of 3-amino-9-ethylcarbazol in 6 ml of dimethylsulfoxide; add, with mixing, to 50 ml of 0.1 mol/L Michaelis buffer, pH 7.4, containing 0.5 ml of 0.3% (w/v) hydrogen peroxide solution. Make up to 100 ml with distilled water.
d. Incubate fixed smear for 15 minutes in the staining solution and rinse in tap water.
e. Counterstain for 10 minutes with Mayer's hematoxylin stain.

Reaction Product.   red-brown; eosinophils, yellow-brown.
Note: Sensitive coloring under immersion oil (which should be removed with xylene). Preparations should be covered.

6.5.3   Sudan Black Stain
(Lison method)

Staining Procedure

a. Stain air-dried preparation in stain-buffer solution.
b. Rinse slide 3 times in 70% (v/v) alcohol until clear.
c. Rinse slide for 2 minutes in running tap water.
d. Counterstain nuclei with Giemsa or Mayers hematoxylin stains.

Reaction Product.   Black, gray-black.

Reagents

Mayer's hematoxylin solution
Giemsa stain
Sudan black B
Phenol
$Na_2HPO_4 \cdot H_2O$

Preparation of Stain Solution

a. Dissolve 0.3 g Sudan black B in 100 ml 100% (v/v) ethanol. Shake well and stand for 2 days at room temperature.

b. To prepare buffer, dissolve 16 g of phenol in 30 ml of absolute ethanol (solution 1). Also, dissolve 0.3 g of $Na_2HPO_4·H_2O$ in 100 ml of distilled water (solution 2). Store at 4° C. Mix 15 ml of solution 1 with 50 ml of solution 2.

c. Mix 60 ml of the Sudan black B solution and 40 ml of the buffer solution. Filter. Stable for 2 to 3 months.

6.5.4   Periodic Acid–Schiff Reaction (PAS reaction)
(Hotchkiss and McManus procedure with the author's modification)

Staining Procedure

a. Fix the slide (bone marrow) for 5 minutes in 10% (v/v) formaldehyde, followed by ether for 30 seconds to remove fat.

b. Rinse the slide in tap water for a short time.

c. Oxidize for 10 minutes in freshly prepared 5 g/L aqueous periodic acid solution. (**Note:** This step must be carried out in the dark.)

d. Wash thoroughly in distilled water.

e. Immerse for 20 to 30 minutes in freshly prepared Schiff's reagent (in the dark).

f. Wash for 10 to 15 minutes under running tap water.

g. Counterstain for 1 to 2 minutes with Mayer's hematoxylin stain.

h. Place under running tap water for 10 minutes to enhance blue color; air dry.

Note: The staining reactions are best carried out on 24-hour-old slides.

Reaction Product.   Crimson red.

Reagents

Methanol

5 g/L aqueous periodic acid solution

Schiff's reagent (see the following for preparation)

Pararosaniline

Potassium bisulphite

Sodium hydroxide

Mayer's hematoxylin solution

Preparation of Schiff's Reagent

a. Dissolve, with shaking, 0.5 g of pararosaniline in 15 ml of 1.0 mol/L hydrochloric acid (solution 1).

b. Dissolve 0.5 g of potassium bisulphite in 85 ml of double distilled water (solution 2).

c. Mix solutions 1 and 2 and stand at room temperature in the dark for 24 hours. Shake well with 300 mg of activated charcoal; then filter.

6.5.5   Cytochemical Iron Determination
(Prussian blue reaction with author's modification)

Staining Procedure

a. Prepare technically perfect slides of marrow smears and touch preparations; air dry.
b. Fix slide for 5 minutes in methanol; air dry. (Slides that are several years old can still be stained by the cytochemical iron reaction.) Remove fat by immersion in ether for 30 seconds.
c. Stain for 5 minutes with acid potassium ferrocyanide solution.
d. Rinse 3 times with distilled water.
e. Stain the nuclei for 1 to 2 minutes with Mayer's hematoxylin stain.

Reaction Product.   Blue.

Reagents

10 g/L potassium ferrocyanide solution; stable for 2 to 3 months stored in a brown glass bottle

37% (concentrated) hydrochloric acid

Staining Solution.   Immediately before the staining, add 0.5 ml of concentrated HCl to 50 ml of 10 g/L potassium ferrocyanide solution.

6.5.6   Acid Phosphatase Reaction
(Löffler method)

Staining Procedure

a. Use air-dried slides less than 8 days old.
b. Fix for 30 seconds in cold (4° C) 60% (v/v) acetone. (Unfixed preparations give the best results.)
c. Wash in tap water.
d. Prepare staining solution:
   (i) Mix 0.4 ml of 4 g/dl pararosaniline solution and 0.4 ml of 40 g/L sodium nitrite solution; allow to stand for at least 1 minute. Dilute the yellow pararosaniline hexazonium salt solution with 30 ml of Michaelis buffer, pH 7.62, and adjust the pH to 5.0–5.1 with 2 mol/L hydrochloric acid.
   (ii) Dissolve 10 mg of naphthol-As-Bi-phosphate in 2 ml of dimethylsulfoxide.
   (iii) Pipet solution 4(i) into solution 4(ii), stirring during addition.
e. Place the slides in the staining solution and stain for 4 hours at room temperature.
f. Rinse thoroughly with tap water.
g. Stain the nuclei with Mayer's hematoxylin stain for 8 to 10 minutes.
h. Allow to develop for at least 15 minutes in running tap water, followed by air drying.

Reaction Product.   Orange–deep red.

Reagents

Acetone 60% (v/v)

50 g/L pararosaniline solution

40 g/L aqueous sodium nitrite solution

Michaelis buffer, pH 7.62

Naphthol-As-Bi-phosphate (store at $-20°$ C)

Dimethylsulfoxide

Mayer's hematoxylin stain

6.5.7   Acid Phosphatase Reaction with Tartrate Inhibition

Staining Procedure

a. Carry out steps a) to c) for Acid Phosphatase Reaction (see p. 115)

b. Mix 0.4 ml of 40 g/L pararosaniline solution with 0.4 ml of 40 g/L sodium nitrite solution; allow to stand for at least 1 minute. Dilute the resulting light yellow pararosaniline hexazonium salt solution with 30 ml of Michaelis buffer. Dissolve 225 mg of tartaric acid in the mixture, and adjust the pH to 5.0–5.1 with 1 mol/L sodium hydroxide.

c. Carry out steps e) to h) of the Acid Phosphatase Reaction (see 6.5.6).

Reagents.   Same as those for Acid Phosphatase Reaction (6.5.6), with L-(+)-tartaric acid.

6.5.8   Acid-Esterase Reaction
(Cottier method)

Staining Procedure

a. Dissolve 10 mg of α-naphthol acetate in 0.4 ml of acetone.

b. Mix 1.2 ml of 40 g/L pararosaniline solution and 1.2 ml of 40 g/L sodium nitrite solution; allow to react for 1 minute.

c. Add 40 ml of pH 5.8 Sörensen buffer to the mixture prepared in step b, and bring to pH 5.8 with 1 mol/L sodium hydroxide solution.

d. Filter the solutions prepared in steps a, and c, into a staining trough.

e. Place the air-dried smear in the solution and incubate for $2\frac{1}{2}$ hours.

f. Rinse with water.

g. Stain for 2 minutes in Mayer's hematoxylin stain.

h. Place under running tap water for 10 minutes to enhance blue color.

Reaction Product.   Coffee brown.

Reagents

α-Naphthol acetate (store at $0°$ C)

40 g/L pararosaniline solution

40 g/L sodium nitrite solution

Sörensen buffer, pH 5.8

Mayer's hematoxylin solution

6.5.9   α-Naphthylacetate Esterase (Nonspecific Esterase) Reaction
(Löffler method)

Staining Procedure

a. Use thin air-dried slide preparations (not more than 8 days old). Fixing the slides in formaldehyde for 5 minutes is not necessary.

b. Place the slide in the staining trough.

c. Mix 8 drops of pararosaniline solution and 8 drops of sodium nitrite solution; allow to react for 1 minute.

d. Add 80 ml of pH 7.0 phosphate buffer to the mixture prepared in step c,

e. Dissolve 20 mg of α-naphthyl acetate in 2 ml of acetone; add (with stirring) the solution prepared in step d, to this solution.

f. Filter the solution prepared in step e, into the staining trough containing the slides. Stain for 30 minutes at room temperature.

g. Rinse carefully under tap water for 10 minutes.

h. Stain with Mayer's hematoxylin stain for 3 minutes.

i. Place under running tap water for 10 minutes to enhance blue color; air dry.

Reaction Product.   Brown–reddish brown.

Reagents

40 g/L pararosaniline solution
40 g/L aqueous sodium nitrite solution
Phosphate buffer, pH 7.0
Acetone (analytic reagent grade)
α-Naphthol acetate
Mayer's hematoxylin solution

6.5.10   Dipeptidylaminopeptidase (DAP IV) Stain
(Lojda and Feller method)

Staining Procedure

a. Fix the slide for 4 seconds in fixing solution (1:10 solution of 10% [v/v] formaldehyde and 90% [v/v] ethanol).

b. Place the slide in the staining solution for 45 minutes.

c. Rinse for 10 minutes under running tap water.

d. Stain for 1½ minutes with Mayer's hematoxylin stain.

e. Rinse for 10 minutes under running tap water.

Reaction Product.   Brick red.

Preparation of Staining Solution

a. Dissolve 7.5 mg of glycyl-L-proline-4-methoxy-β-naphthylamide in 1.0 ml of dimethyl formamide; add 20 ml of 0.1 mol/L phosphate buffer, pH 7.0. (Solution 1, sufficient for 2 slides.)

b. Dissolve 20 mg of fast-blue B dye in 1 ml of dimethyl formamide (solution 2).

c. Mix solutions 1 and 2, then filter.

Preparation of Buffer Solution (pH 7.0)

a. 0.1 mol/L $Na_2HPO_4 \cdot 2H_2O$, 35.814 g/L (solution 1).

b. 0.1 mol/L $NaH_2PO_4 \cdot 2H_2O$, 13.799 g/L (solution 2).

c. Mix 660 ml of solution 1 with 340 ml of solution 2; check pH 7.0 with a pH meter.

6.5.11   Toluidine Blue Stain for Basophils
(Undritz procedure)

Reagent.   Saturated toluidine blue in methanol. Dissolve 1 g of toluidine blue in 100 ml of methanol (very stable).

Staining.   Simultaneously fix and stain the air-dried smear by placing the slide in a staining tray and pouring the toluidine blue-methanol solution over the slide. Rinse with running tap water and air dry.

Result.   The granulation in blood or bone marrow basophils is stained red-violet as a result of the strong metachromic effects of heparin sulphate.

Index

Page numbers in *italics* indicate illustrations; numbers followed by "t" indicate tables.